# SIMPLE
# ELECTRONIC
# NAVIGATION

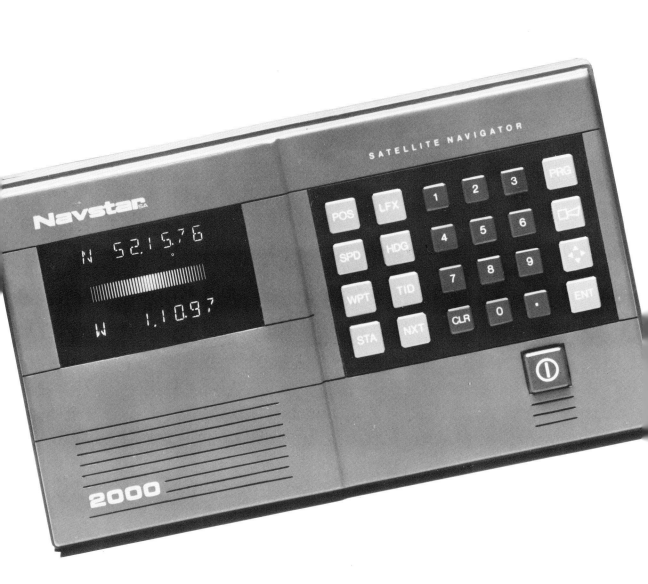

# SIMPLE
# ELECTRONIC
# NAVIGATION

## Mik Chinery

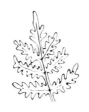

## Fernhurst Books

© Fernhurst Books 1988

First published 1988 by Fernhurst Books,
33 Grand Parade, Brighton, East Sussex
BN2 2QA

Chinery, Mik
    Simple electronic navigation.
    1. Boats and ships. Electronic navigation
equipment
    I. Title    II. A Yachtmaster's guide
    623.89 3

ISBN 0 906754 67 4

## Acknowledgements

The publishers would like to thank Bill Anderson of the RYA for
his detailed comments on the manuscript, and Roger Shannon
and the staff of Navstar Ltd for supplying technical information.

The Admiralty charts reproduced on pages 47 and 48 are
Crown Copyright, reproduced from Admiralty charts with the
permission of the Controller of Her Majesty's Stationery Office
and of the Hydrographer of the Navy.

The charts on pages 43 and 44 are reproduced with the
permission of Barnacle Marine Ltd, and the chart on page 45 is
reproduced with the permission of Imray Laurie Norie & Wilson
Ltd.

## Photographs

The photographs in this book were supplied by the following:
British Telecom: page 60
Mik Chinery: pages 15, 34
Janet Harber: page 31
Motor Boat and Yachting magazine: pages 7, 9, 11, 14, 22, 25, 28,
30, 32, 46, 49, 53, 57, 58
Navstar Ltd: pages 2, 8, 10, 16, 18, 24, 26
Pickthall Picture Library: pages 19, 55
John Woodward: Front cover

Design by John Woodward
Artwork by PanTek, Maidstone
Cover design by Behram Kapadia
Composition by Book Economy Services, Burgess Hill

Printed and bound by World Print Ltd in Hong Kong

# Contents

You do not need to know anything about crankshafts and pistons to learn how to drive a car. In the same way, you do not have to be an expert in radio wave propagation and electronic engineering to learn how to use an electronic navigator. Accordingly, in this book the theory behind the various systems is described only briefly, in the final chapter.

If anyone is to blame for this book it is George Taylor, the editor of *Practical Boat Owner* magazine. He suggested it – and he promised to buy the first copy!

**Mik Chinery**

# 1  Introduction

It is a common complaint that in these days of microchip technology the owners' handbooks supplied with most items of electronic equipment are written by experts, for experts. Marine electronic equipment is no exception, and this book is designed to unravel some of the mysteries surrounding the use of electronic navigation devices. It will tell you, in simple terms, how to get the best out of the systems and make them work for you.

The advent of electronic position finding equipment has enormously simplified the routine of navigation at sea, but it should not be relied on exclusively, and must not be considered a substitute for traditional methods of navigation. Indeed, a thorough knowledge of traditional methods of navigation will enable an operator to get much more out of the electronics than someone with limited knowledge. All the techniques should be used together, but although electronic navigators are often considered to be little more than navigational aids it will not be very long before the instruments and methods of traditional navigation are regarded as the aids and the electronic system becomes the norm. How many of us would go to sea without the box of electronics we call an echo sounder? How many of us still carry a leadline and a tin of tallow?

RDF (radio direction finding) has been deliberately omitted from this book for two reasons: there are several excellent books on the subject already, and with stations gradually closing down around Europe it will inevitably become the poor relation to the more modern equipment – which not only provides greater accuracy but has more information to offer than a simple bearing line.

▷ **Signs of the times: the nav. station of transatlantic challenger *Gentry Eagle* is equipped with a whole arsenal of electronic navigation systems.**

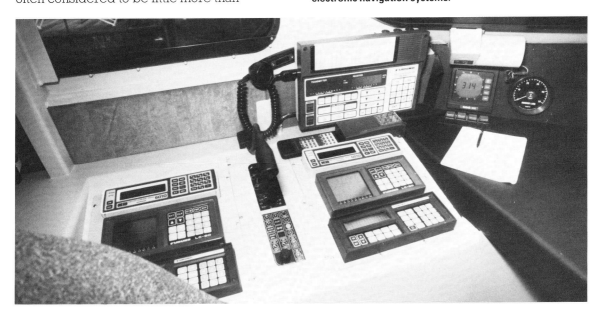

# 2 Choosing a set

A glance through the window of your local marine electronics dealer will reveal a bewildering array of electronic navigators employing a variety of systems. Decca, Loran C and Transit; there are examples of each type available with a vast price range extending up to the price of a luxury car. Very few of us have unlimited finances, so it is just as well that the most expensive is not necessarily the most suitable for our purposes.

In order to choose the right set the first question you have to ask yourself is 'Where do I anticipate doing my boating?' The answer to this question could mean that you need two navigators, each using a different system, to cover all the areas you plan to sail in. So let us consider the options available.

## DECCA

The Decca navigation system covers all of northern Europe with excellent coverage in Scandinavia and the Baltic area and reasonable coverage in the western Channel. The coverage extends south down the Portuguese coast and around to Gibraltar but does not extend into the Mediterranean. There are other Decca areas around major ports in the world such as parts of Australia and Japan, but the best-served areas are confined to northern Europe. Having the advantage of continuous fixes every few seconds Decca has become the leading system in Europe for private and professional users.

The UK government wishes to introduce a Loran C system to replace the British Decca chains which they are planning to phase out

during 1997. Despite this the Scandinavian countries have recently invested large amounts of money in their Decca systems to bring them up to date. They have no plans for the introduction of a Loran C system. If the UK government are unable reach International agreement to introduce Loran C to Europe by the end of 1991 then the only alternative is to update and renew the British Decca chains. Either way the Decca system will continue to operate at full efficiency in UK waters until 1996.

## LORAN C

This American system operates at greater ranges than Decca, so the Loran stations on the north-east coast of America, together with stations in the far north of Norway, can give continuous cover across the northern Atlantic. The coverage is good in Scandinavia, but moving southward the transmissions become very thin on the ground south of Scotland and there is no cover for the southern North Sea or

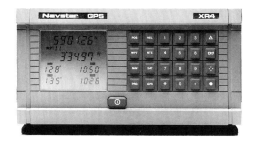
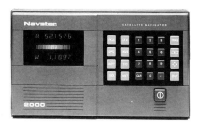

◊ Finances permitting, you should buy the set that is best suited to your type of sailing. Here a GPS set (top) is shown with a less expensive Transit Satnav.

the western approaches. However, Loran C owners are catered for in the Mediterranean where a series of stations gives reasonable operation over the whole of the region.

## TRANSIT AND GPS

The Transit Satnav system gives world-wide coverage, but has the disadvantage of giving only about 30 fixes every 24 hours with 'fix gaps' of up to four hours. This is not a problem for the deep-sea ocean navigator, but if you are rock-hopping around the north Brittany coast the Transit system is of little use. The GPS or 'Global Positioning System' is a more advanced satellite system which, when it is fully operational, will give continuous fixes anywhere in the world. Undoubtedly this is the ultimate system, but there are two drawbacks.

The first is that owing to setbacks in the American space shuttle programme the system has still not been completed. It is unlikely that the full satellite 'umbrella' to give 24-hour coverage will be in operation before 1992. Currently (1990) the coverage is around 22 hours per day but this fluctuates as some satellites are turned on and off for adjustments. The other drawback is the cost, since even the cheapest GPS receivers are at least three times the price of a Decca or Loran set. As GPS sets have more complicated and therefore more expensive technology it is unlikely that prices will fall to compare with Decca or Loran units.

## CONCLUSION

As mentioned earlier, you could buy two navigators to cover your requirements. Maybe you intend to sail part of the season in northern Europe and part in the Mediterranean; in this case you could justify buying both a Decca and a Loran C set. Perhaps you normally sail in the Med and intend to cruise across the Atlantic to the Caribbean; to do this you may want to have a Loran C set and a Transit Satnav receiver or a GPS set for the deep-sea navigation. In the end it comes back to the original question 'Where do I intend to take my boat?' and with GPS over the horizon you might add 'How much do I want to spend?'

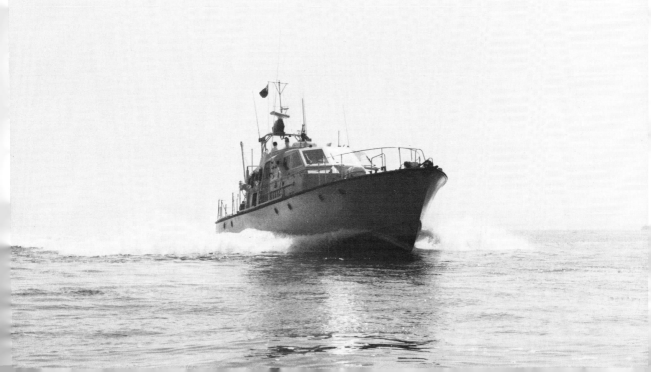

# 3   Installation: Decca and Loran C

It is worth taking a lot of care when installing your new navigator. The most expensive machine may give suspect information if it is badly installed, and a navigator that gives wrong information is worse than useless. By following a few simple guidelines you can be sure of getting the best from any machine.

## MOUNTING POSITION

When you are deciding on a mounting position for your navigator you have to take three things into account. First, what type of display does it have? Second, is it waterproof? Third, where is the helm position?

### Display
The models with LEDs (light emitting diodes) such as Navstar, Walker, and the Shipmate 4000 series are almost impossible to read in bright sunlight, so if your unit has one of these displays it should be mounted inside, in a shaded spot.

LCD (liquid crystal display) types such as AP, Decca, Shipmate 4500, Raytheon and the Navstar 2000L are equipped with a device to increase their image contrast in bright light. These sets are obviously more suited to the brighter mounting positions. At night both types work well: the LED types all have dimmer settings to reduce glare and the LCD types are softly backlit with red or green light.

### Waterproofing
The waterproofing of any piece of electronic gear is always suspect. Most navigator manufacturers describe their equipment as 'splashproof' – which means that it will not stand regular dowsing with salt spray. Waterproof housings can be obtained for many of the popular navigators; these are guaranteed to be spray- and wave-proof.

▽  **This Loran C set has an LCD read-out that is legible in bright sunlight.**

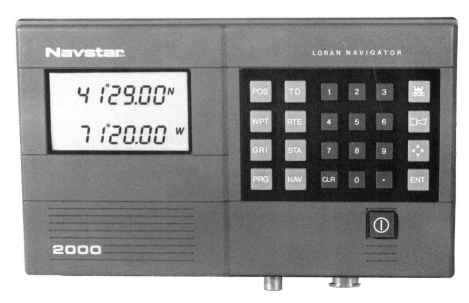

### Helm position

An added complication affecting the choice of a mounting position is the need to mount the display close to the helm. On a fast motor cruiser the helmsman may be steering by cross-track error and will need to look at the display every two or three minutes. Similarly, on a sailing boat on a short reach across the tide the helmsman may prefer to steer by watching the cross-track display. In both circumstances it does not help if the set is mounted down below in the navigator's position, or on the opposite side of the saloon to the helmsman.

One solution is to use a repeater instrument. These are available for most sets, and consist of separate display units which are waterproof and can be cockpit mounted. The more sophisticated models are active; that is to say they have simple controls to select display information from the navigator.

However, on long sailing trips where the tide is expected to vary or turn during the passage, the helmsman steers to a compass course dictated at intervals by a real (human) navigator. Under such conditions the electronics are best situated down below.

## POWER SUPPLIES

Electronic navigators take very little electrical power, but the wires supplying this power must be thick enough to avoid voltage drop. This is particularly important in the case of a satellite navigator, which has a very accurate internal clock that is temperature stabilised to ensure synchronisation with the transmission signals. The correct temperature is maintained by housing the clock in a miniature electric oven.

Although the power consumption is small it may still be significant for a yacht on a long ocean passage. Practical experiments have shown that solar charging panels, propshaft alternators and wind chargers in conjunction with a battery can operate most electronic navigators almost indefinitely without any problems. Modern navigators are all equipped with cut-off circuits so that in the event of falling battery voltage the set will switch off before there is any possibility of false information being displayed.

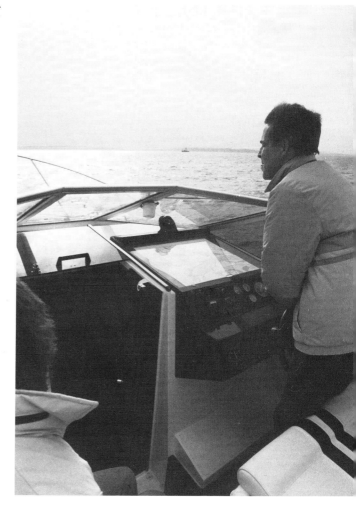

◊ **Cockpit mounting can be a great help to the helmsman – but make sure the machine is waterproof!**

To minimise shipboard electrical interference it is advisable to take power direct from the ship's battery via a separate fuse link. Further protection from interference can be obtained by using twin screened cable, with the outer braided screen connected to earth via the hull ground plate, keel or P-bracket bolts.

## AERIAL POSITION

Many owners go to a great deal of trouble and expense to mount their Decca/Loran aerials on top of the mast, but in many cases a high mounting does not guarantee the best performance. A more important contribution to good aerial performance is what the experts call 'ground plane'; in simple terms this means making a good electrical contact with the water surface so that it acts as a reflector for radio signals. The easiest way to ensure a good ground plane effect is to earth the fixing point of the aerial base to a hull ground plate. On sailing boats mounting the aerial on the stern pushpit rail will generally give good results, but further improvements to reception can be obtained by earthing the rail. A wire connected from one of the fixing bolts down to an earthing point can sometimes increase signal strength by as much as 20 per cent.

Aerial mounting positions to avoid are: mounting inside the framework formed by rigging such as the triangle between forestay, mast and backstay; close to another aerial or vertical metal object such as a mast or section of wire rigging; or alongside a metal-framed windscreen or canopy frame.

◊  **On a sailing yacht, the highest aerial position is not necessarily the best.**

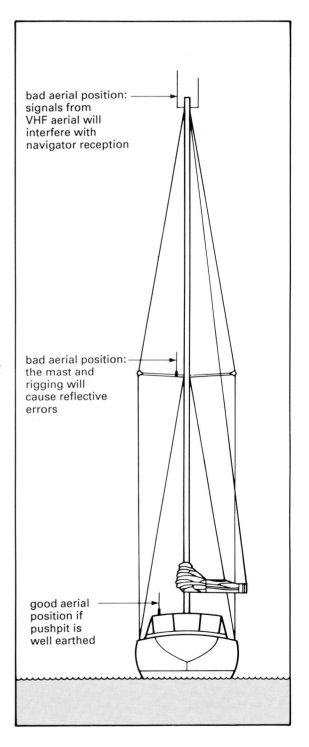

bad aerial position: signals from VHF aerial will interfere with navigator reception

bad aerial position: the mast and rigging will cause reflective errors

good aerial position if pushpit is well earthed

If the aerial is mounted in one of these positions it can cause an error on some ship's headings. For example, if the navigator is displaying a distant point as a bearing, aerial shielding can cause an apparent 'bending' of the displayed bearing by as much as five degrees.

The following simple check will show up any shielding problems. Enter the latitude and longitude of a distant waypoint (see chapter 5) into the machine. Make sure that the waypoint is more than 100 miles away from your position and then call up the distance and bearing display. Start the boat's engine and motor round in a tight circle while watching the waypoint bearing. As the ship's head rotates, any aerial shielding problems will cause the waypoint bearing on the display to flick up and down a few degrees. If you have a shielding problem then move the aerial around the boat, mounting it temporarily with adhesive tape, to find the best position. When you find a position that allows you to rotate the boat without any change in the bearing of the distant waypoint, then make the aerial a permanent fixture.

Make sure that the aerial is as far away from the VHF radio antenna as possible; at worst they should be no closer than two metres apart. If the aerials are too close together severe interference may be experienced when the VHF transmit button is pressed. If you ever find yourself using the VHF to transmit the dreaded words 'Mayday, Mayday, Mayday; this is yacht *Dingbat, Dingbat, Dingbat*; my position is . . .' it will not help much when you look at the navigator to find that your transmission has wiped out the display! To check for this find an unused VHF channel, make sure the set is switched to 25 watts output, then press the transmit key while watching the signal strength display on the navigator (see overleaf).

The ships's radar installation should not cause any problems with your Decca/Loran set provided the aerials are not mounted on the 'sweep' line of the radar scanner. Some navigator aerials have sensitive electronic circuits which are easily and irreparably damaged by direct radar waves at close range, so always ensure that your Decca/Loran aerial is above or below the horizontal line extending from the radar scanner unit.

▷ **The aerial will work much better if it is properly earthed. Here the pushpit rail is earthed to a metal ground plate bolted to the hull.**

▷ **Mounting the aerial in the signal path of a radar scanner can irreparably damage the navigator, so raise it clear on a mast or framework.**

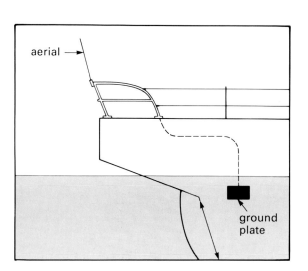

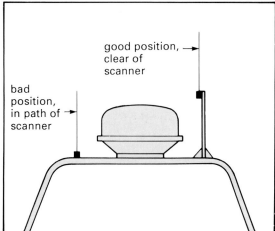

## ELECTRICAL INTERFERENCE

Many owners of electronic navigators complain of intermittent operation: 'It works fine for a couple of hours, then it goes haywire', or 'My set does not work in the rain'. In nine cases out of ten these complaints can be attributed to on-board electrical interference of some kind.

All electronic navigators have a signal strength display in the form of four readings showing the signals received from the land stations. Most of the displays use a 0-9 scale, zero meaning a bad signal and nine signifying a good signal. One exception to this rule is the AP/Decca MK 4 which reverses the score: zero is good and nine is bad! To check your installation for electrical interference call up this display on the unit, then go around the boat switching on every electrical appliance in turn. Wait at least one full minute after switching on each item, and watch the signal strength display. If the figure gets worse then you have some electrical interference.

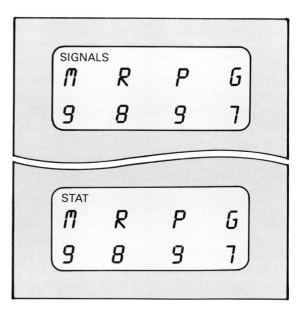

▷ Two types of signal strength display, showing the strength of signals from the master station and the 'red', 'purple' and 'green' slave stations.
▷ If a navigator on a motor boat stops working in the rain it is probably suffering from interference generated by the windscreen wipers!

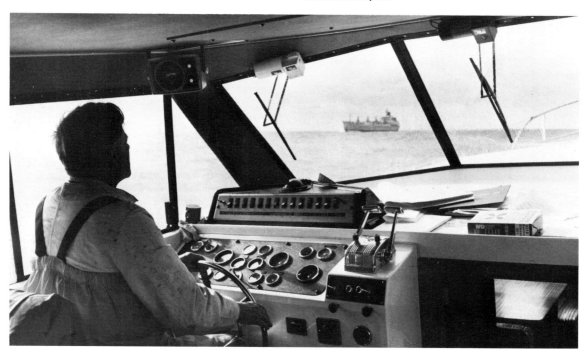

The sources of interference that are hardest to find are the things we do not use very often. For example, navigators that do not like the rain are usually being sabotaged by windscreen wipers. Navigators that play up every couple of hours are probably listening to the on-board refrigerator, which only turns on now and again. Automatic bilge pumps are another source of intermittent electrical noise. One case that the author investigated involved a set that lost its memory and position every time the skipper's wife used the toilet! The WC was a manual pump model with no electrical parts and when other members of the crew used it there was no problem with the navigator. After many frustrating hours the solution was found: the skipper's wife always turned on the light in the toilet, but nobody else bothered. The light fitting was one of the popular low-voltage fluorescent fittings manufactured in the Far East. These fittings can sometimes radiate enough interference to affect every piece of electronic equipment on board.

Fish-finder echo sounders of the graphic display type can sometimes cause severe interference and loss of signal if they are wired to the same power supply as the navigator. The simple answer here is to wire each set to the ship's battery independently.

Engines can interfere with electronic navigators in several ways. The first is when you start the motor and the display wipes out, only to reappear a few seconds later as the set relocates itself. This phenomenon is caused by voltage drop while the engine's starter motor is operating. It does not harm the electronics but it can be frustrating and perhaps dangerous to lose the set for a few minutes while it updates and settles down. The best cure is to have independent power supplies for the engine and other ancillary circuits. Simple blocking diodes can be fitted to enable the two batteries to be charged from one alternator while remaining electrically independent from each other when supplying power.

Another prime source of engine interference is the alternator charging system. Some improvements can be made by fitting suppression capacitors to the alternators, and your marine engine agent will give individual advice on this problem. In the writer's experience automotive suppressors of 1 or 3 microfarad rating are not sufficient. In some cases large capacitors of up to 15 microfarad rating have proved very successful in difficult situations.

If you experience severe electrical interference problems with your set then a final solution is to install a separate battery as the sole supply for the electronics. The power consumption of an electronic navigator is very low and an average-sized car battery will operate a set for several days. When the battery is low it can be connected into the ship's charging system for a top-up.

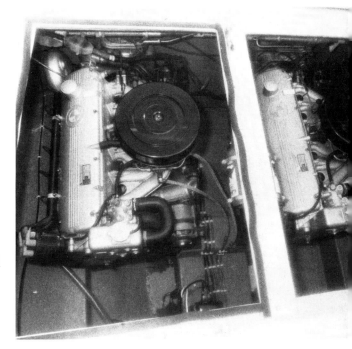

◊ **Engines are a major source of interference. If the usual suppressors don't work you may need to run your navigator off a completely separate power supply.**

## INTERFACING

Given the quantity of information an electronic navigator can provide it seems wasteful not to make the most of it. One way of utilising the set's potential is to interface – that is connect it to another device that can use the navigation data it is producing. The simplest interface is to connect a printer to give a printed output of information at a regular time interval. Unfortunately not every set has the built-in software for this; at the time of writing the only machines that can drive a printer are the Shipmate models, the Navstar 603 and 2000 units, the AP/Decca 5, Magnavox and Trimble sets.

Autopilot interfaces are now becoming very popular. With this connection the ship can be kept on a strictly controlled course to a waypoint with little or no deviation either side of the track line. The navigator automatically takes into account the variables such as tide and leeway and sends information to the autopilot, which then steers the ship straight for the next waypoint.

A track plotter – which is essentially an electronic chart displayed on a TV-type screen – has to be driven by a navigator; it can show your track and intended course on the screen together with any waypoints within range of the screen display selected.

All of these devices have to be connected via the correct interface. Most modern sets have the interface software built in, but you have to buy a separate unit for many older sets. Such units are so expensive that it is often cheaper and better to replace the whole navigator with a new machine – which will offer many extra facilities besides built-in interfaces.

Unfortunately there are several different types of interface, each with its own number. To drive a printer you must have a set with an RS232 output; all other types of interface are covered by the following numbers: NMEA180, NMEA182 and NMEA183. The more sophisticated sets have them all built in, and

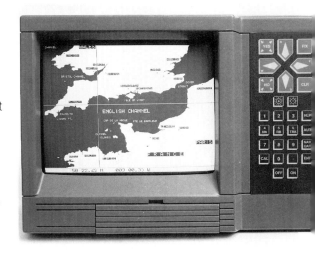

⟡  **By linking a track plotter to your navigator, via the appropriate interface, you get an instant picture of your position and progress projected on an electronic chart.**

you can select the one you want from the keypad. It is important to select the best one for your purpose, but do not despair; any competent marine electronics dealer will be able to unravel the mysteries of interfacing your particular installation.

There is one major difference between these interface numbers. NMEA180 and 182 come to almost the same thing in performance terms but NMEA183 is substantially different. If you connect an electronic navigator to an autopilot using either of the interfaces 180 or 182, the set will direct the autopilot to steer to the next waypoint. When the boat reaches the waypoint the navigator is automatically disconnected from the autopilot, which then keeps the boat running on the same course until the pilot is turned off or the course is changed.

If you are using the NMEA183 interface between your navigator and pilot then things happen differently. When the boat reaches a waypoint the navigator switches to the next one on the route; the autopilot may change course accordingly and start steering for the next waypoint. This situation will continue for as long as the navigator keeps supplying new waypoints. The danger is that you could enter a route into your navigator, start off, then go below for a cup of tea or, worse, a few hours' sleep while leaving the electronics to run the ship. Interfacing can be a very useful and worthwhile exercise but it must be used with a large dose of common sense.

Another item that can be added to your navigator via an interface cable is the Yeoman chart plotter system. The unit consists of an electronically active plastic membrane half the size of an Admiralty chart and an electronic 'puck'. An ordinary chart is clipped behind the membrane and, once three points are co-ordinated, the puck will give instantaneous lat/long readings as it is moved around the chart.

When the system is interfaced with the navigator, indicators on the puck light up to show the way it has to be moved to coincide with the ship's position. This makes it easy to plot your position on the chart. Waypoints can be uploaded directly from the chart to the navigator, and bearings, distances and tracks can be easily measured. The system is simple and accurate and can be operated by less experienced crew members who may have limited knowledge of navigation.

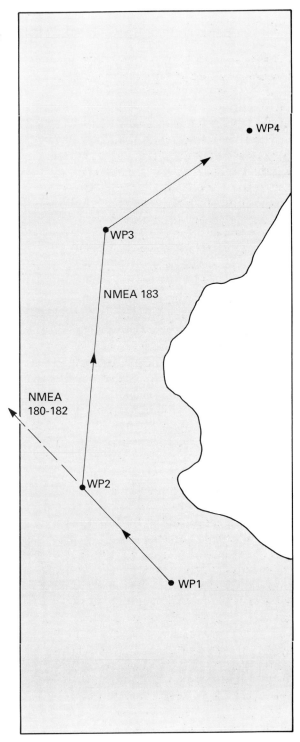

◊ **If you link an autopilot to your machine via an NMEA 180 or 182 interface the boat will steer itself to a waypoint, but it will keep the same course beyond the waypoint until it is redirected. If the navigator is fitted with an NMEA 183 interface and switched to 'Pilot' mode or its equivalent, it may switch itself to the new course automatically and the autopilot will follow suit to steer the boat along the whole route.**

# 4 Installation: Transit and GPS

Satellite navigation systems rely on transmissions from satellites passing overhead in pre-determined orbits. Since the signal is coming from high above the horizon the aerial height is not important, but as with the other systems you must take care to avoid any shielding by metal structures, rigging and spars. It is possible to mount the aerials inside the saloon and still get good results, but as before the favoured position is on the pushpit, which should be earthed to the water via a ground plate. Masthead fixings are fine provided that care is taken to keep the aerial away from the VHF aerial. Satellite systems work on much higher frequencies than Loran or Decca so the aerials are short and stumpy and convenient to mount almost anywhere. Another advantage of the higher frequencies is that they reject almost all electrical interference from on-board systems.

⬦ **GPS sets use stumpy aerials that can be mounted almost anywhere on the boat.**

## CALIBRATION

The GPS Navstar system works at very high speeds with position updates every few milliseconds, so heading and speed information is not required. On the other hand speed and heading information (and height of aerial) is fundamental to the operation of the Transit system. It also takes several minutes to calculate a fix, so this extra information is needed to allow the machine to apply a correction to the last fix and give a D R (dead reckoning) position. This position is only as good as the information that is entered into the computer so if you are beating to windward with varying speeds and headings the Satnav is going to have a hard time. The best way to eliminate these sources of error is to fit heading and speed reference units that will give the electronic navigator constant information and eliminate the need for operator input. Trials have shown that a Transit receiver, fitted with such units that have been checked and calibrated, can give constant position displays accurate to within 250 metres.

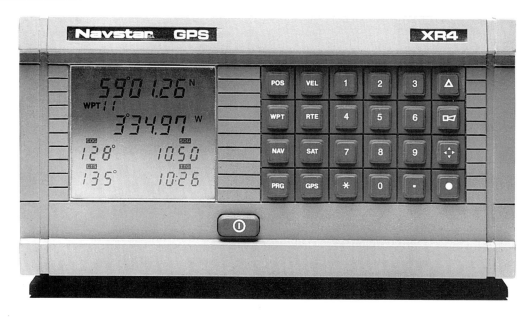

To achieve this standard of accuracy from the set the heading reference unit (which is a compass) has to be accurately swung by an experienced compass adjuster unless it is a self-calibration type. These sophisticated units require the helmsman to steer the boat around in a steady circle while the software in the compass works out the deviation errors and stores them in memory. This procedure can usually produce a heading reading accurate to within a couple of degrees.

The speed sensor (which can be the transducer of the ship's log) has to provide accurate information on distance travelled. You can adjust it yourself if you have the patience to spend a day going up and down a measured mile to calibrate it. Electronic log sending-units output their information in pulses of electricity: a certain number of pulses per mile. The precise number can usually be found in the log instruction book. Since the Satnav can be adjusted to receive any number of pulses per mile, you can tune the system for accuracy. To start with, enter the number of pulses that the log manufacturer recommends (a common figure is 1000 pulses per mile). Set the navigator display to show speed in knots, then motor up and down your local measured mile. Take a mean time for the two-way run and work out your true speed. If this does not correspond to the reading shown on the Satnav then alter the pulse figure up or down and make a repeat run up and down the mile. Using this method, you can adjust the speed input so the error is less than two per cent.

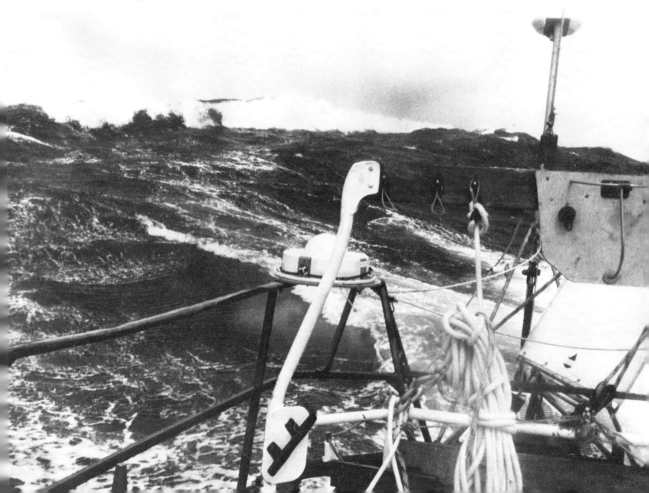

▽ **Heavy weather in the Southern Ocean. It is here, well beyond the range of the Decca and Loran C chains, that the Satnav systems come into their own.**

# 5 Initial programming

Irrespective of make, all electronic navigators require very similar basic information to be programmed into them when they are first installed. Once this has been done the internal lithium batteries will retain all the information in the memory for three months or more, regardless of whether the set is used, and switching on recharges the batteries for a further three months or so.

Provided the set is switched on before you move away from your berth and switched off when you leave the boat the unit will track your position at all times. But if you forget to turn the set on it may lose itself unless it is equipped with an autolocate facility. This is rather like blindfolding somebody and taking him for a car ride before releasing him: he will have problems re-orienting himself to the new surroundings until you give him a clue.

The autolocate feature on a Decca set should overcome this problem, but it is not foolproof. Some units autolocate by listening into two Decca chains, but if you are in a fringe area the signals from the second chain may be too weak, so the system fails to work. Another autolocation system requires you to enter your estimated position and a radius of possible error. This

⇨ **If you forget to turn your set on when you leave your home berth it may get lost. If you turn it on at point A it will be fine, for it is still within a three-mile radius of the starting point, but at point B it is out of range. It will need a new position to within three miles; here the beacon on the island would do, but the church on the shore is too far away. A rough fix (using a transit of the two crossed with the heading from the harbour) would be a more seamanlike solution.**

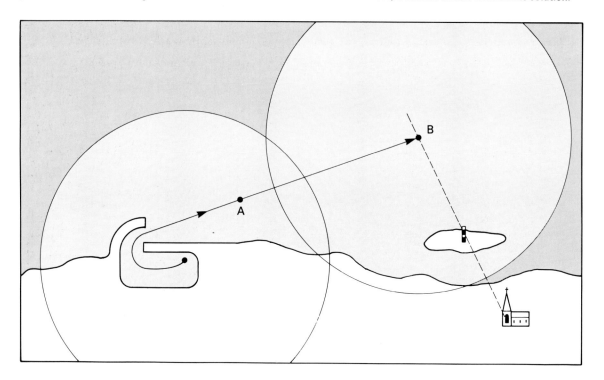

should enable the set to lock on correctly, but there are occasions when it may fail. All in all it is much better to make a habit of turning the set on before you leave your berth.

### Date and time

Date and time sound straightforward but can be confusing; this is because dates are displayed in alpha numeric, but have to be entered in numeric form. Depending on the set some require English date format and others require American. For example, 15th July 1989 would be displayed as 15 Jul 89 but would be entered as 150789 (or 071589 on some machines). The time entry is easier – just four figures are needed, despite the fact that the display shows hours, minutes and seconds. Two-thirty in the afternoon would be entered as 1430, and would be displayed as 14.30.00. With Loran C and Decca sets the time entered can be your local time or whatever time reference you are using to navigate with. A satellite navigator needs to have GMT (Greenwich Mean Time) or UTC (Universal Time Co-ordinate) entered to an accuracy of within ten minutes; after one or two satellite passes the set will correct the time itself to within a few milliseconds.

### Start position

The initial start position needs to be known within three miles and has to be entered as a latitude and longitude reading. Here we encounter the most common operator error: the east-west problem. When you enter the latitude and longitude of a position or waypoint into a navigator, the set will assume that the latitude is northerly and the longitude is easterly. This is fine if you are off the coast of Norway, but will be very confusing if you are off southern Ireland! In such circumstances you must enter *westerly* latitude by pressing the plus/minus

◊ **If you are sailing west of the Greenwich meridian (or south of the equator) be sure to double-check all your lat/long positions.**

key. Even the most experienced users of marine electronics make this mistake occasionally, so the rule is to check and double-check after you have entered any lat/long co-ordinates.

A Navstar satellite navigator has an auto-locate facility; if the GMT time is entered correctly to within 10 minutes the machine will find itself – anywhere in the world. This is especially useful for the long-distance yachtsman who has limited power available: the set can be turned on for an hour or so every 24 hours to receive a fix, then switched off to conserve power.

### Variation and deviation

On most electronic navigators magnetic variation can be entered so that all bearing displays show magnetic readings. A variation of five degrees 20 minutes west would be entered as 05.20, pressing the plus/minus key for west. This can be useful, but beware of this feature if

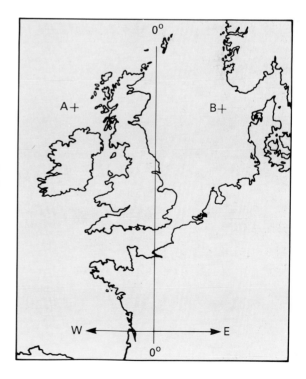

you go on a long cruise away from home, for the same variation will be applied until you change it. For example, if you sail from the south coast of England to the Brittany coast of France the variation you experience changes by more than two degrees. Ocean-crossing yachtsmen can experience changes in variation of up to 15 degrees in 1000 sea miles. So remember to update the correction figure as you move into a different area.

The Shipmate 4000 sets do not have correction for variation and read only in degrees true. At the other end of the scale the Navstar 2000 series Decca, Loran and Satnav machines have an automatic variation feature. When programming the 2000 you have a choice of true or magnetic bearings. If you choose magnetic, then the display instantly shows the variation for your area. The software works out the figure by using the position information relative to the month and year, so magnetic bearings are displayed correctly at all times irrespective of your position.

The Navstar 2000 series and the Philips AP5 can also accept deviation in 45-degree segments and will interpolate between these points to give bearings and courses to steer that are corrected for the ship's compass. If this information is entered the effect can be confusing, for if you decide to check the bearing of a visible waypoint with the handbearing compass the figure you come up with may not match the course to steer indicated by the navigator. If this happens, try aiming the boat at the waypoint: the figure on the steering compass (which is suffering from the deviation programmed into the machine) should match that shown on the electronic navigator. If it doesn't, the deviation figures must be wrong.

**Chain search**

Once the set has been told the date, time and estimated position it will search for the nearest group of transmitting stations (the chain) and lock on to their frequencies, giving a position fix

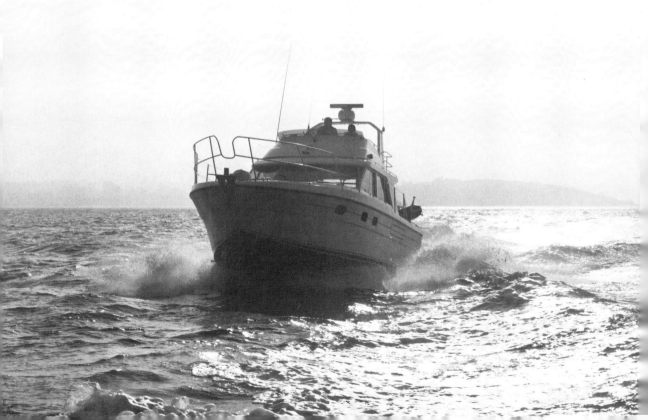

lock on to their frequencies, giving a position fix after two or three minutes. This chain search is automatic and the set will choose the chain giving the best signals for your area. If the vessel moves out of range of the chain first selected, then the set will simply choose another that is within range and continue operating.

## ALARM FUNCTIONS

All manufacturers include alarm functions on their sets to give audible and visible warnings of problem areas. On start-up the unit goes through a self-test routine checking the receiver, the software and the aerial connections. If it finds fault with any of these tests an alarm is activated. Other alarms include low battery voltage, no position update, lost lock LOP (line of position) error, off-course alarm, anchor watch alarm, signal suspect, third slave error, closest point of approach to waypoint, satellite fix completed . . . and some even have a built-in alarm clock! Any or all of these alarms can be turned off in the programming stages. In each case the plus/minus key will switch between yes or no each time an alarm page is shown on the display.

### Waypoint alarm
The waypoint alarm deserves a special mention, since it can perform two functions. When you are setting up your electronic navigator and dealing with the various alarms the set will request 'Waypoint alarm yes/no?' Pressing the plus/minus key will select the answer, and if you enter 'Yes' the set will request a distance. The figure you now enter is the distance you want to be from a waypoint

when the set bleeps at you to remind you of the fact. For most purposes a figure of 0.2 miles is appropriate. Key this in, and the set will draw an imaginary circle with a radius of 0.2 miles around each waypoint. When the boat enters this circle from any direction the alarm is activated.

This is straightforward enough, but the other function of the waypoint alarm is less obvious. The waypoint alarm distance also controls the automatic switch-over from one waypoint to the next in the sequence or route. If you have

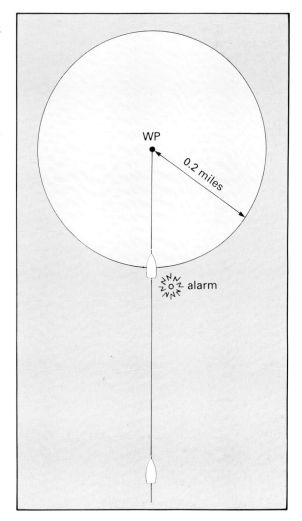

◊ **By setting the waypoint alarm you get audible warning that you are nearly there – and also trigger the machine to switch to the new waypoint.**

entered a route into your set as a sequence of waypoints, you expect to sail from one to the other in the same sequence. When you arrive at each waypoint you can manually enter the identifying number of the next, and the heading information will appear on the display. If the 'Route', 'Pilot' or 'Sailplan' facility is used, however, then on arrival at a waypoint the set will automatically switch to the next, assuming the waypoint alarm is turned on and the distance set is not too small. Otherwise the auto switching will not take place and you will have to enter the number of the next waypoint manually.

## PRINTED RECORDS

Some electronic navigators have an RS232 output facility to operate a small printer. This can be a useful safety feature, especially if the set can be programmed to automatically print

information at regular intervals. For example, a regular printed record giving position, time, course made good and distance to the next waypoint would be invaluable if the electronics were to fail for any reason. If your set has the facility, you can enter the time that you would like each print-out to appear. For sailing boats a print-out every 30 minutes is enough, but skippers of faster-moving motor cruisers should be looking for a print-out every 15 minutes or so. The choice of suitable printers is very restricted and at the time of writing none of the manufacturers offer a printer as an accessory. The printer needs to have RS232 input and operate on a 12-volt supply. One inexpensive model that works well in most applications is the Epson P40. This is a thermal transfer unit that prints up to 40 characters wide on a continuous roll of paper.

▷ **Today many boats use on-board computers, and you can now buy a GPS receiver that slots into the PC.**

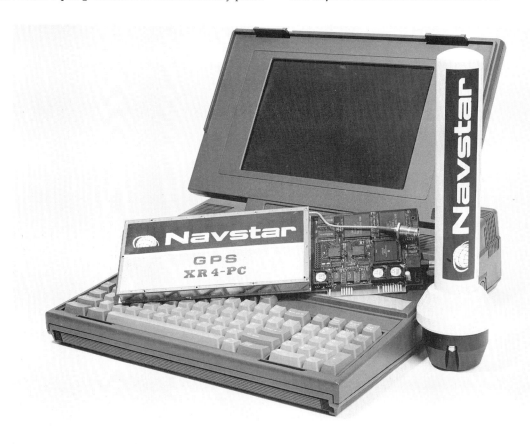

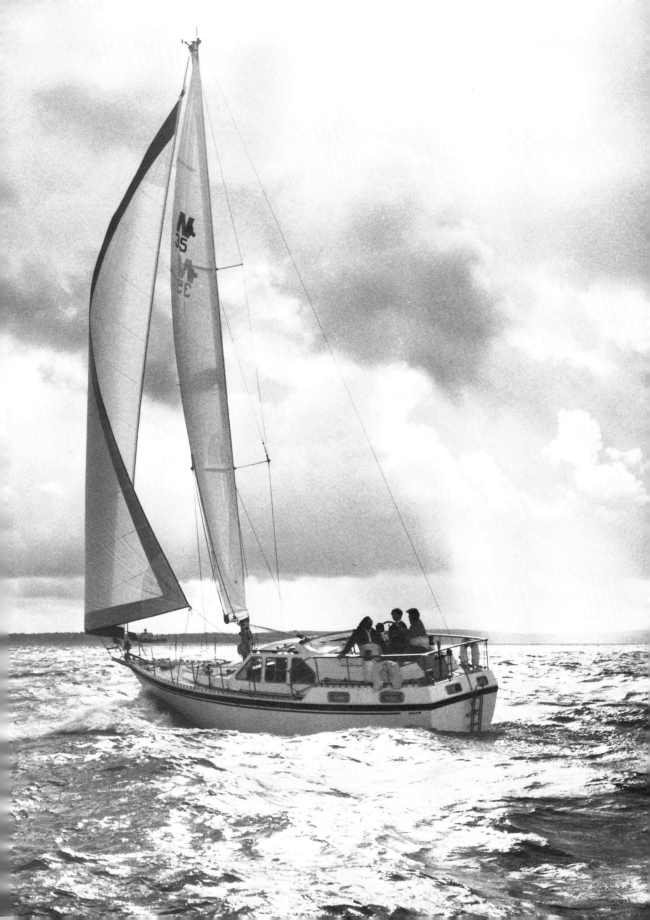

# 6 Simple outputs

Most of the basic information you need from your navigator is available at the press of a button.

## POSITION

The simplest output from a navigator is the ship's position in latitude and longitude, which you obtain by pressing the POS button. On Loran and Decca units this information is updated every five seconds or less on recent sets, and every 20 seconds on older models. GPS sets update in less than one second but Transit Satnav sets receive only about 30 fixes a

⬡ **The most basic output: a lat/long position displayed on a Decca navigator in degrees, minutes and decimals of a minute.**

day. These fixes are memorised and most units will show the last 12 fixes (some store 20 or more) giving the time, the position in lat/long and the grade of fix. They can also work out the times of future fixes so you know when the next one is due. In between these fixes the Transit sets make use of a DR (dead reckoning) system; this requires speed and heading information, but will keep the position display updating.

## SPEED AND COURSE

With Decca and Loran C, pressing the VEL (velocity) button will display SMG (speed-made-good) or SOG (speed-over-ground) depending on which set you have. This is an

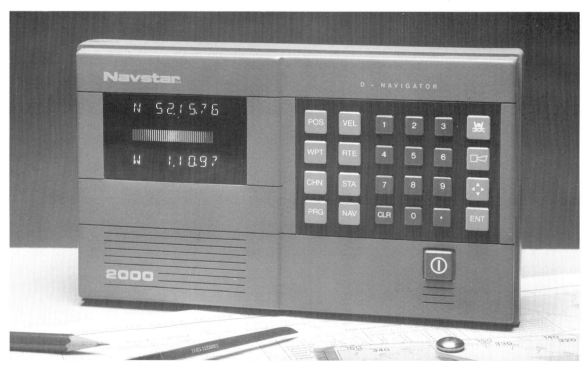

accurate measurement of your true speed over the seabed irrespective of tide or wind. Another push of the VEL button will show CMG (course-made-good) or COG (course-over-ground). As with the speed display this is the course you are achieving over the ground irrespective of the effects of tide or wind. These two figures can be used to check on the amount of compensation that you are applying for tide, wind and leeway. Checking the displayed speed against the ship's log will show the difference between actual speed and speed through the water. The difference between the course-made-good reading and the ship's compass heading shows the course offset caused by leeway, and tidal stream.

> In this cross-tide, the COG (course-over-ground) and SOG (speed-over-ground) displays show the actual course and speed, so there is no need to draw tidal vectors on the chart. By making allowance for the drift by steering 10 degrees up-tide, the helmsman can bring up the correct course on the COG display (000 degrees) and make straight for the waypoint.

## SIGNAL STRENGTH

Pressing the STA (status) button will show the relative signal strengths being received from the master and slave stations. Readings are on a 0-9 scale with zero being bad and nine being excellent (except for the AP/Decca Mk 4 model which reverses the score).

## RANGE

The time to waypoint can be shown as hours and minutes or, for long-distance sailors, a time and date. To take this feature to extremes the effect of increasing or shortening sail on your intended arrival time can be seen instantly by looking at your electronic navigator. Distances can be displayed in RL (rhumb line) or GC (great circle) routes for long-distance sailors and it is simple to switch between the two to see which is appropriate.

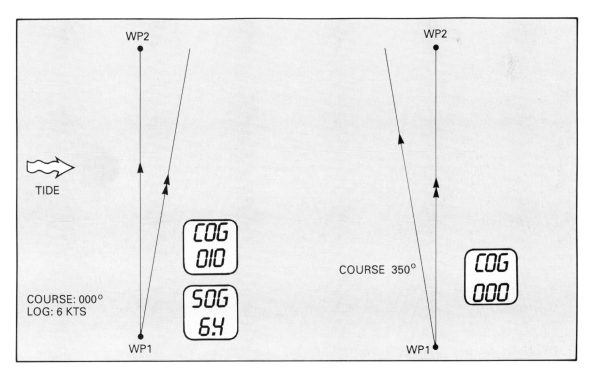

TIDE

WP2

WP1

COG
010

SOG
6.4

COURSE: 000°
LOG: 6 KTS

WP2

WP1

COURSE 350°

COG
000

# 7   Waypoint sailing

A waypoint is simply a point you wish to sail to. It can be a buoy, a harbour entrance, an anchorage, a point off a lighthouse, a point off a headland or just a position at sea. Whatever it is, you need to know its position in degrees of latitude and longitude so it can be entered into the machine. If you are entering a series of waypoints, which may be your route to a favourite destination, then make a list of the positions, in order, on a waypoint sheet. A copy of a waypoint sheet can be found in the back of this book. Do not write on this one; use it as a master for making photocopies.

Fill in the location of the waypoint, the lat/long position, and the bearing and distance from the start position or previous waypoint. All this information can be derived from your chart.

## ENTERING THE WAYPOINTS

Having filled in your waypoint sheet, you are ready to enter each position into the navigator, taking special note of the east/west notation on the longitude. You will probably enter the waypoints in the order that you are intending to sail along them, but this is not essential.

Next decide on a route, which is simply the order in which you want to proceed along the list of waypoints. Some sets refer to a route while others call it a sailplan or pilot plan. The Phillips AP sets have an auto sailplan function. This works by automatically forming a route of waypoints as you enter each one into the set.

⊘   **An unmistakable seamark such as this LANBY makes a perfect waypoint, for it allows you to check the performance of the navigator and adjust the lat/long co-ordinates of the waypoint to give maximum accuracy in the future.**

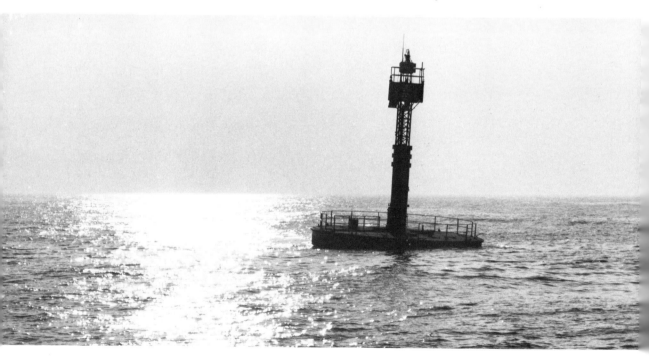

This is fine until, at a later date, you wish to return home along the same route. Then you have to turn off the auto sailplan function and re-enter the waypoint sequence in reverse order. If you have one of the Shipmate navigators then a reverse route is no problem; at the touch of a button the machine reverses the pilot plan, as it calls it, and you can return along the sequence of waypoints.

## SETTING OFF

Once you have your waypoints entered into the navigator you can set off from your berth towards waypoint one. The internal computer will draw an imaginary line between each point on the route, but remember that this line is the shortest distance between the two points and is drawn irrespective of any land or other obstructions appearing in between! To enter the waypoint sailing mode you have to press the WPT button on Navstar-style sets or 'Navigate' on Decca sets. Subsequent presses of the button will show distance and bearing to waypoint, time remaining to waypoint, and cross-track information.

The cross-track information is the real heart of the system. The set will show both in distance, and graphically, how far to one side of the ground track between two waypoints you are. For example, if the tide has pushed you off course to starboard the display could show a row of arrowheads pointing to port and a figure of 1.2 miles. This means that you are a little over one mile off course to starboard, and the arrowheads are indicating that you should steer to port to compensate for the error.

Here the cross-tide has pushed the boat 10 degrees off course. By checking the cross-track display at point A the helmsman can see that he is 1.2 miles off track, and has to steer to port. The display also gives him the bearing and distance to the waypoint from his current position.

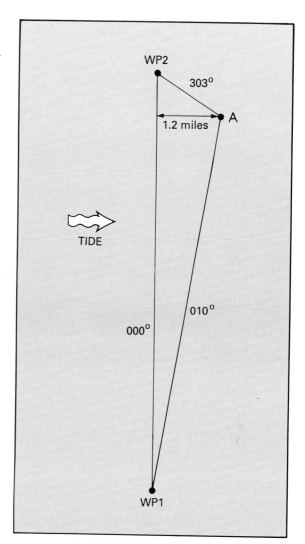

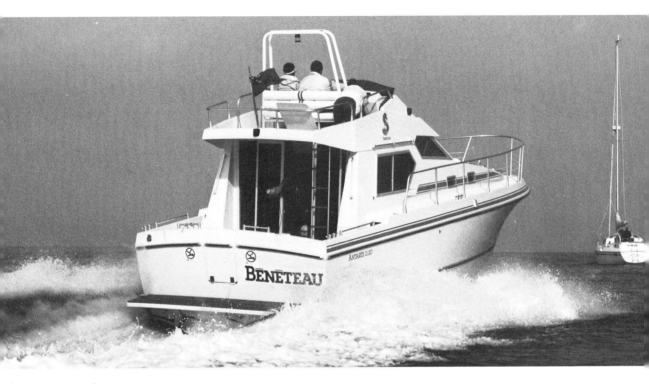

This system of steering the boat takes into account all the possible variables which could affect your course accuracy, such as tide and wind. You might think that it requires constant course alterations, but in practice a sailing boat normally needs only slight course adjustment every half hour, while a faster power boat may need an adjustment every 15 minutes. If your navigator is interfaced with an autopilot then the course will be adjusted automatically so that the vessel sails straight down the ground track. Whether this is appropriate for your sailing strategy is another matter, and we will look at the advantages and disadvantages of steering by cross-track error in chapter 8.

Most electronic navigators can accept information on tide direction and speed. For Loran C and Decca owners this is only of use if you are using the internal computer as a dead reckoning calculator to work out an initial course to steer. For normal navigation this data is not required as it is a simple matter to steer a

⌁ **Even a fast motor boat can be given its head for 15 minutes or so before increasing cross-track error dictates a slight course alteration.**

direct course to the next waypoint and watch the cross-track error. Within two or three minutes the increasing error one way indicates a change of course, and then the optimum heading can be maintained to stay on track. Another method is to note the bearing of the waypoint, then look at the course-made-good or course-over-ground displays. The difference between the two bearings is the amount of compass offset required to keep the vessel on track. Always bear in mind that the cross-track information that the machine gives is not dependent on knowing the tides or winds; it reduces these variables to a simple cross-track error measurement which is easily correctable by the helmsman. But when using a satellite navigator the tide speed and direction must be entered to enable the set to operate, and work

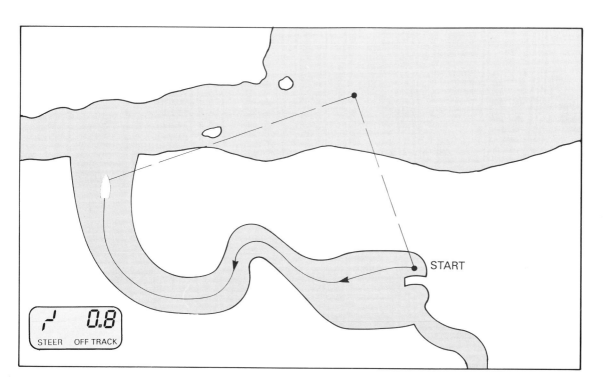

out DR (dead reckoning) information between fixes.

## STARTING ERROR

One area of confusion encountered when waypoint sailing is the apparently large cross-track error experienced when you are on the way to waypoint one. One fact that is rarely made clear in the instruction books is that the start-up position of the set is considered to be waypoint zero, so the computer will draw an imaginary line between the start position, which could be your marina berth, to the first waypoint you entered. A straight line from your berth to waypoint one will almost certainly cross over land or other obstructions, so if you have motored out from your mooring into the fairway and clear water then you will be some way off the first track – and the error will be shown on the display.

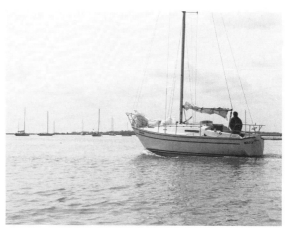

◁   **As you motor out of harbour the navigator will try to direct you overland to the first waypoint. Here the display is indicating a 0.8-mile cross-track error and suggesting a change of course to starboard, which is not much help.**

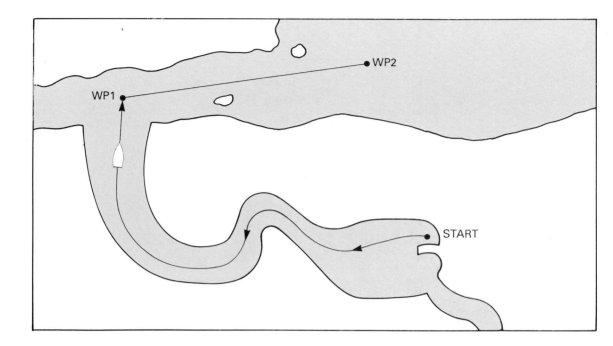

If visibility is poor then you need to have accurate cross-track information as you travel to waypoint one. What is needed is for the set to re-draw the imaginary line from your present position in the fairway to the first waypoint. One method is to re-enter the boat's position on the program, but this is tedious and mistakes can be made. The more seamanlike method is to include another waypoint in your route, at the entrance to your river or fairway, but if you have a limited number of waypoints available on your machine there is a quick way to get it to re-draw the imaginary line from your position to the next waypoint. Just turn the navigator off and on again, so it is forced to re-calculate its position. All the initial information will be intact, since the internal battery ensures that all such data is stored. Within a minute or so the set will show zero cross-track error and will direct you to the next waypoint without any problem. The Navstar 2000 machines employ an even simpler method for re-setting the cross-track error: you just press the zero key followed by the enter key to bring the figures back to zero.

▱ There is little you can do about the passage down the meandering channel, but by entering another waypoint in the fairway you can use cross-track information to avoid the rocks on the way out to the open sea. This could be invaluable in a fog, or at night. By switching the machine off and on again once you are in the fairway you can achieve much the same result, since the navigator will take 'WP1' as its starting position.

▱ You probably navigate your home waters by eye – but remember that a few waypoints stored in the machine may come in very useful when the visibility drops to a few feet.

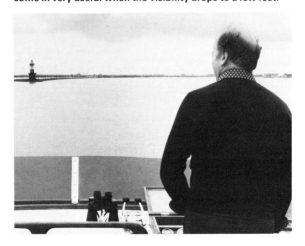

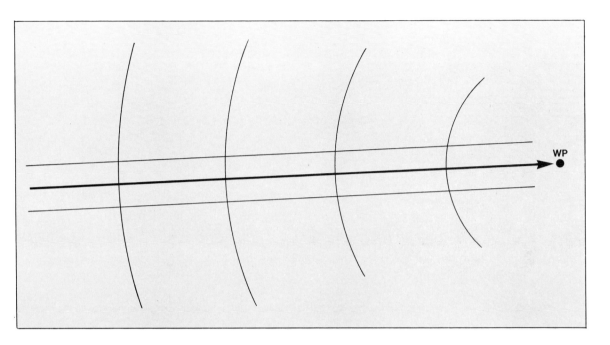

## PLOTTING YOUR POSITION

The other essential part of the waypoint display is the bearing and distance reading to the next waypoint. It is very important that regular positions are plotted as the boat moves along. Many people take the position readings in lat/long and mark the spot on the chart every so often. This is laborious and sometimes difficult to do on a small boat that is rolling about. A simpler method is to note the bearing and distance from the waypoint to give a chart fix. This position is exactly the same as the lat/long reading because both figures are derived from the same source of information. Another benefit of this is that if you are following the cross-track information and steering without any errors, then a fix requires just a distance measurement marked off the course line on the chart.

It is very useful to mark the chart in advance with distances from a waypoint, using a pair of compasses to scribe short arcs at regular intervals along the route – say every five miles on a long voyage. When you are on passage

◁ By marking distances from a waypoint as arcs crossing your intended track on the chart, you can rapidly plot your position. Here the display shows that you are 16.5 miles from the waypoint with a 0.3 mile crosstrack error to port. The arcs are at five-mile intervals, with 'corridor lines' one mile each side of the track. Where are you?

you can see at a glance approximately where you are by taking the distance-to-go reading from your navigator and applying it to the chart.

## ARRIVAL TIME

The ETA (estimated time of arrival) at the waypoint is displayed in different ways depending on the set. Shipmate sets show a time of arrival and the date. Navstar sets show hours and minutes while Decca units give arrival time but no date. Other timing functions can include a countdown alarm for racing, an alarm clock and an average speed and distance calculation. This will show the average speed plus total distance run since the counter was last set to zero.

Decca Range
450m day
250m night

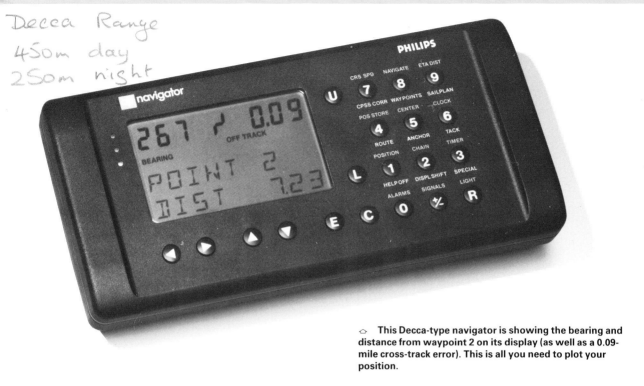

⇧ This Decca-type navigator is showing the bearing and distance from waypoint 2 on its display (as well as a 0.09-mile cross-track error). This is all you need to plot your position.

## ACCURACY

There are certain fixed errors in the Decca system of radio transmissions, but the system can be operated to accuracies of 200 metres or less under most conditions. In real terms this means that you can enter a waypoint position derived from a chart and expect to come within 200 metres of it. In practice the author has rarely found any errors greater than 100 metres when approaching a strange landfall. For Loran C users the error figures are greater, but accuracies of 800 metres or less can be relied upon under most conditions of good coverage. Repeat readings taken when returning to the same spot are usually within 200 metres or less. Larger errors may be experienced with both systems, but these are usually found some distance offshore or in fringe reception areas that are known well in advance.

The Loran C system may be less accurate than Decca, but the reception range plus coverage areas are greater. The Decca system covers most of northern Europe but does not extend more than 50 miles or so into the Mediterranean from Gibraltar. Loran C covers most of the Mediterranean and the north Atlantic areas between Norway and Canada and extends down the eastern seaboard of the USA.

To get the most accurate results you must use the repeat factor. By this method you can use Loran C in the Mediterranean to achieve accuracies of 150 metres or so, and in northern Europe Decca can be used to give positions accurate to within 30 metres. To get this degree of precision you have to note down the lat/long position the set is giving when you are at an identifiable waypoint. If you use the same waypoint in the future you enter the lat/long position you noted when last there, instead of taking it from the chart. If this technique of 'using the reading when last here' is used the system can be relied upon to give consistent, repeatable results.

## RECORDING WAYPOINTS

The waypoint sheet supplied with this book has been designed for the purpose of recording position readings at each stage. When you reach each point on the sheet, note the reading of the set, the ship's log reading and the time. This not only records the position for future use but gives a fix to return to if the electronic systems fail at any time. The sheets can be collected in a ring binder for future use; we are all creatures of habit and we all tend to return to our favourite sailing waters from time to time.

Sets with large waypoint memories can be filled with positions, all or some of which can be combined to give a route at any time. Multi-waypoint machines also enable you to record your turning points and channel information back into harbour and on to your mooring or marina berth. On more than one occasion the author has returned across the English Channel in perfect conditions only to encounter a thick fog in the Solent. Normally when this happens the ship's navigator must rush to the chart and work out a series of waypoints back to the berth. This is the time when haste may lead to mistakes when transposing a list of lat/long figures from the chart to the electronic equipment.

To avoid this possibility it makes good sea sense to check out the courses and turning points into harbour and back to your own berth before you have to do it for real. Pick a day with good visibility, start from your berth and go to each turning point on your way out, taking a position reading each time. Store the readings on a waypoint sheet, but also keep them in the navigator's memory for when they are needed. When the day comes that you have to find your way back home in the dark or a thick fog you will have all the positions easily to hand and will be able to get back to your berth safely.

If you have a Navstar 2000 set things are a little easier when it comes to recording position readings. When you are in a spot you wish to record you press the WPT key followed by the POS key and the waypoint number. The set files the present position in that waypoint slot for future use. Other sets can be operated in a similar manner but use a more complicated key function.

The system of recording positions for future use is of enormous value and should be maintained. When you enter a harbour, no matter how well you know it, take a position reading at the entrance and note it down on a waypoint sheet. The next time you visit the place it could be in thick fog. Be sure to take the position reading between the entrance walls and not alongside one of them, or you could hit the wall on a future visit. The positions you note throughout a season will work consistently and accurately on your boat in the future. They will not work on another boat, though, particularly if it has a different make of navigator and installation set-up, so your sailing friends cannot borrow your waypoint sheet and copy your positions for their own use.

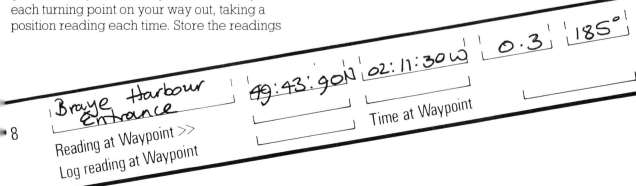

# 8   Refinements

Once you have grasped the principles of using waypoint navigation coupled with cross-track information there are many ways the system can be used to improve your boating.

## TIDAL STREAMS

When you use traditional methods of navigation on a cross-channel voyage you may well allow yourself to be swept to one side and then back again by the tidal flow in both directions. This way your vessel will sail or motor along the route between two points and cover the shortest distance *over the water* despite being swept to one side for some of the time and back again for the remainder.

If you were to try and cover the shortest distance *over the ground* by sticking to the direct line drawn on a chart and using the cross-track information on your box of electronics, then you would cover a greater distance through the water – so it would take longer. As an extreme example, consider a 60-mile crossing of the English Channel in a boat making five knots, and experiencing a six-hour flood tide followed by a six-hour ebb tide. The passage time would be 12 hours, and if the tide velocity was a steady 1.5 knots, and traditional methods were used to take advantage of the tide, the total distance travelled would be 60 miles. If the electronics were used to follow a direct line with tide compensation all the way the distance travelled would be 2.5 miles longer or 0.5 hours extra sailing time. In a light wind the extra sailing time would increase dramatically. But if the boat's speed was 10 knots and the start time was delayed to allow three hours' tide one way and three hours' tide the other way, then by following the direct line – electronically – the extra distance travelled

would be less than 0.25 miles. In other words the journey would take 1.5 minutes longer.

The message is clear. On a slow boat – and this includes most sailing boats – it pays to use the traditional methods to save sailing time. On a fast boat, following the direct line with the aid of the cross-track display will still result in a longer passage, but the difference may not be significant enough to justify working out all the variables of tide and wind.

By using the cross-track displays and sailing down the direct line between two points these variable factors are automatically taken into account. The electronic navigator is only interested in your position relative to the sea bed and will clearly show if you are being pushed off course, in any direction, from the ground track between your start position and the next waypoint.

## BEATING TO WINDWARD

Obviously there are some situations where a sailing boat cannot sail down a line because of head winds, and has to beat at about 45 degrees to the wind to make any headway. If you are a long way from your destination the cross-track error figure can be used to indicate when you should tack. For example, if the wind is on the nose your tacks will be roughly symmetrical about the wind direction. Select a distance, say five miles, then sail until your cross-track error is showing five miles. Go about and sail on the other tack; the error will reduce to zero then start to increase as you cross over your course line. When you reach a five-mile error the other side of the line go about again, and so on.

If the wind is off the bow but you still have to beat, then ignore the rhumb line and draw a

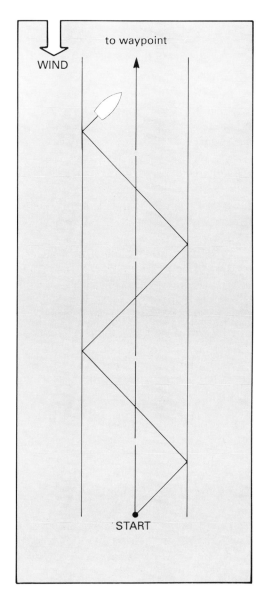

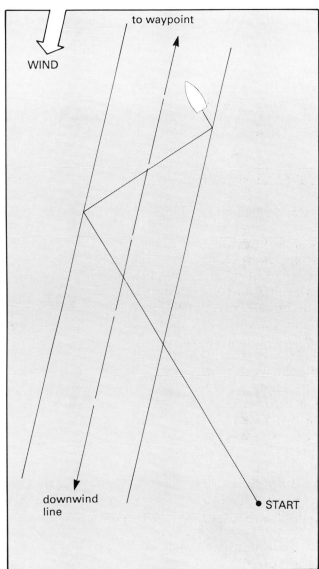

line on the chart directly down wind of your destination. Set up, say, five-mile parallels either side of this line and beat between them. Both examples are ways of making your own set of parallel lines that you can tack between while still maintaining the correct, average heading.

when beating to windward (left) you can set up parallel guidelines either side of your course to the waypoint and use the cross-track information to tell you when to tack. If the wind is off the bow you simply re-lay the course and guidelines so they bear directly downwind of the waypoint, then keep sailing until, as before, the cross-track error indicates that it is time to tack.

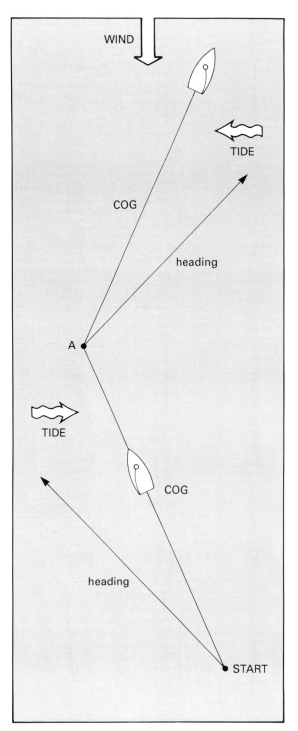

However, Decca does not have all the answers: don't forget the tide. When beating, sail as much as possible with the tide on your lee bow (see diagram). By careful tacking you can ensure that the tide lifts the boat to windward on each tack.

### Closer to home

When you are getting closer to the waypoint, within say ten miles or so, it can be difficult to judge the last few tacks to ensure that you arrive exactly on target and not downtide. The way to deal with this problem is to choose a 'target' a sensible distance uptide of your destination. Then draw a line directly

◊ ◁ **By beating into the tide (left) and tacking when the tide turns you can get the current to 'lift' you towards your destination. Get it wrong (below) and you get nowhere, slowly. Note that the compass heading is the same in both examples, but the COG display will tell you if you have made the right decisions.**

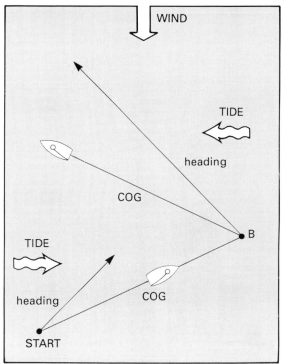

downwind of your target and construct a 60 degree cone (2 × 30°) about the downwind line. Make sure there are no dangers within the cone, then note the bearing of each boundary line. Now you can switch your attention from the cross-track display to the 'bearing of waypoint' display. In our example we have drawn two lines each at 30 degrees to the downwind line. So each time we see one of the bearings indicated on the set we can go about and start another tack. This tack is maintained until the display shows the other bearing, at which point the boat is put about again, and so on.

So on a long trip with head winds you can tack between two parallel lines either side of the course until you are eight or ten miles away,

depending on conditions, and then use the two-bearing method to sail up a 'funnel' to the waypoint. Remember that this method takes into account all the variables such as tide, leeway, boatspeed and the numerous course changes you make while sailing the boat at the optimum angle to the wind.

◊ ▽ **When you get near your goal, draw bearing lines on the chart that clear all dangers, note them down, and watch the 'bearing to waypoint' display as you beat upwind. Go about every time one of the bearings comes up on the machine, and you will find yourself tacking down a 'cone' to your destination (left). If the wind is off the bow, draw a downwind line from the waypoint and use this as the basis for the bearing lines (below).**

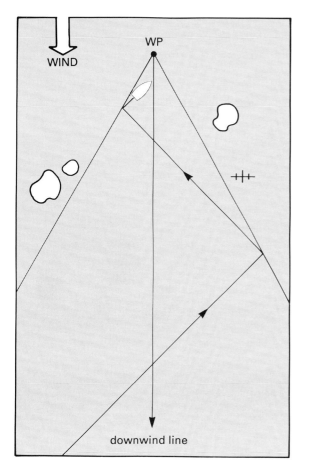

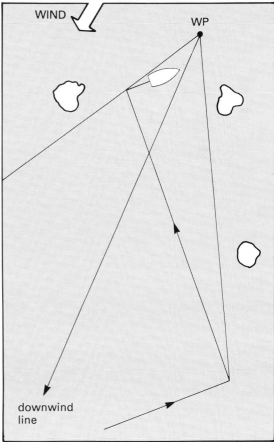

# 9   Making a trip

Let us take a closer look at an actual voyage from the Hamble River on the south coast of England to St Peter Port in Guernsey, via Alderney. Since this is a comparatively short cruise we will be using a Decca-type navigator or GPS set, since the Transit Satnav system with

its 30 or so fixes a day would not prove very effective.

## PLANNING

The first step of any voyage, and sometimes one of the most interesting, is to open up the charts and pilot books to decide where to go. It is at this stage that we determine our route and pick the best positions for use as waypoints. This part of the operation can be carried out at home in the comfort of your armchair, and if you have a suitable power supply for your navigator then the waypoint information can be entered into the machine at the same time. It is not necessary to take the navigator aerial off the boat, because you will not be interested in receiving signals at home (unless you want to plot your house position); just use the memory facility on the unit to store your intended passage. Of course the 'antenna fail' alarm will keep buzzing, so this will have to be turned off to preserve your sanity.

Starting from Hamble Point Marina pick out the selected waypoints on the chart and enter the latitude and longitude of each one, plus the bearings and distances between them, onto the waypoint sheet. Check them carefully and then enter the lat/long into the navigator; the internal battery will preserve the readings until you are ready to install the set back on board and start your journey.

◊   The trip described follows a route from Hamble in southern England, through the Solent and across the English Channel to Braye in Alderney. After an overnight stop in Alderney the route continues to St Peter Port in Guernsey.

◊   The waypoints for the trip, noted on a (simplified) waypoint sheet.

## NAVIGATION WAYPOINT SHEET

**ROUTE:** HAMBLE TO ST PETER PORT

| | DESCRIPTION | LAT. | LONG. | DIS. | BRG. |
|---|---|---|---|---|---|
| **WP1** | HAMBLE POINT BUOY ↓ YB | 50:50:18N | 01:18:58W | 1.0 | 180° |
| **WP2** | CASTLE POINT BUOY Red can | 50:48:68N | 01:17:58W | 1.6 | 156° |
| **WP3** | POINT OFF CALSHOT SPIT | 50:48:33N | 01:17:60W | 0.4 | 180° |
| **WP4** | EAST LEPE BUOY Red can | 50:46:08N | 01:20:85W | 3.0 | 223° |
| **WP5** | N.E. SHINGLES BUOY ◆ BYB | 50:41:94N | 01:33:25W | 9.0 | 242° |
| **WP6** | POINT OFF THE NEEDLES | 50:39:58N | 01:35:88W | 2.9 | 216° |
| **WP7** | POINT OFF BRAYE HARBOUR | 49:44:25N | 02:11:25W | 62.2 | 202° |
| **WP8** | BRAYE HARBOUR ENTRANCE | 49:43:90N | 02:11:30W | 0.3 | 187° |
| **WP9** | POINT IN THE SWINGE | 49:43:30N | 02:14:28W | 2.2 | 252° |
| **WP10** | POINT OFF PLATTE FOUGERE | 49:30:50N | 02:28:50W | 15.7 | 217° |
| **WP11** | POINT OFF ROUSTEL TWR | 49:29:30N | 02:28:90W | 1.2 | 179° |
| **WP12** | ST PETER PORT HARBOUR ENTRANCE | 49:27:40N | 02:31:41W | 2.6 | 222° |

If you have a machine with a sailplan or routing facility you can now enter the passage plan. The first seven waypoints will be passed in number order, and when you arrive at waypoint seven off Braye Harbour, you will turn almost 90 degrees in towards the harbour entrance (waypoint eight). This is obvious, but when you leave the next day to continue your passage you will leave the harbour entrance and sail towards waypoint seven again, the point off Braye. From seven the next waypoint in your passage will be number nine. In short, your route or sailplan would have waypoint seven entered twice. The waypoint sequence will be 1, 2, 3, 4, 5, 6, 7, 8, 7, 9, 10, 11, 12. This allows you to detour off into the harbour and out again the next day without resetting the machine.

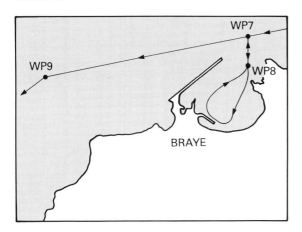

## READY TO GO

With the set back on board and packed with information you are now ready to leave, but before you cast off remember to switch the navigator on and let it settle down for a few minutes. Then plot your position on your local chart, using the information on the display, to ensure that the navigator is working and giving good information. It is good practice to make a note of the latitude and longitude of your home

berth so that you need only glance at the navigator to verify the plot and do not have to transfer it to the chart every time.

Before you leave, select the waypoint or navigate page on the machine and the bearing and distance to waypoint one will be shown on the display. Remember that this bearing is a straight line from your berth out to the Hamble Point buoy so it has to be ignored as you navigate the narrow winding channel. When you arrive at the buoy (waypoint one), take a note of the lat/long reading on the set and note it down in the box on the waypoint sheet for future use.

If you have entered a route plan then the set should automatically switch to the display for waypoint two. If your set does not have this facility then enter waypoint two as the next point to go for. In this example you left at high water, so by now the tide is starting to ebb down Southampton Water. The bearing of waypoint two is shown as 161 degrees, if you steer this course for a few minutes a cross-track error will begin to grow and the arrows will indicate that you should alter course to starboard to compensate for the ebbing tide pushing you off to port. You can alter course by a few degrees and watch the display to achieve an optimum course by trial and error, or you can press the button for COG (course-over-ground). This may show a figure of 155 degrees, a difference from the bearing of six degrees. This means you are being pushed off course by six degrees, so you should now add six degrees to the bearing of 161 to make it 167 degrees; this should give you the correct tide/course compensation for this leg.

On arrival at waypoint three, the point off Calshot Spit, you follow the same procedure to the next waypoint, and so on. After leaving waypoint four, the course takes you along the Solent. If you have set a steady cruising speed of 10 knots then you can press the SOG (speed-over-ground) button to see the actual speed you are making over the ground. On a spring

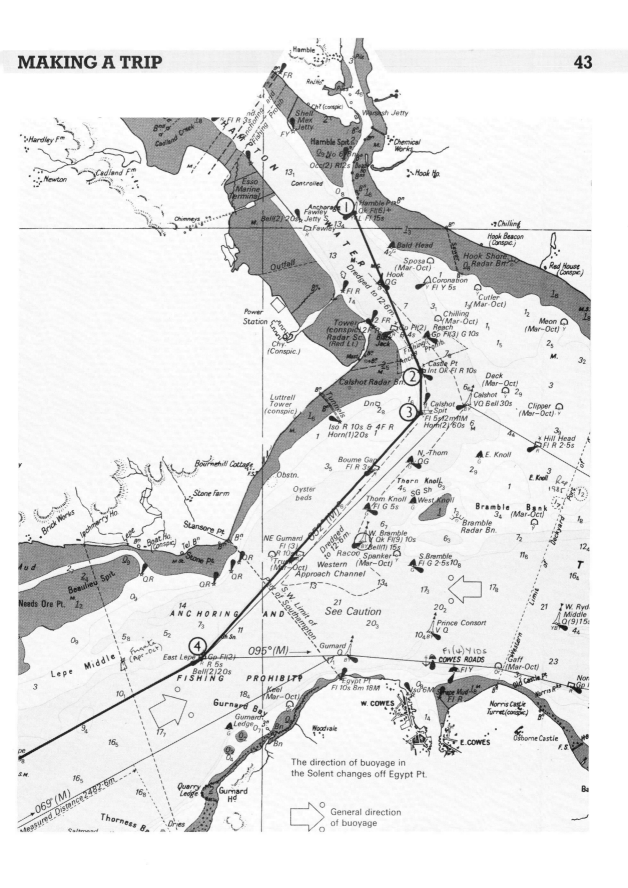

The direction of buoyage in
the Solent changes off Egypt Pt.

General direction
of buoyage

tide the machine may indicate a speed of 12.5 knots, which means that you are gaining 2.5 knots over your cruising speed as the beneficial tide helps the boat along. On this leg the tide may be easing you off course to starboard, but the cross-track display will soon show this up and a slight correction to port will keep you on course for the next waypoint. Remember to note the lat/long reading given on the navigator each time you arrive at a waypoint, together with the time and the ship's log reading, so you have a good fix to work from if the electronics stop working.

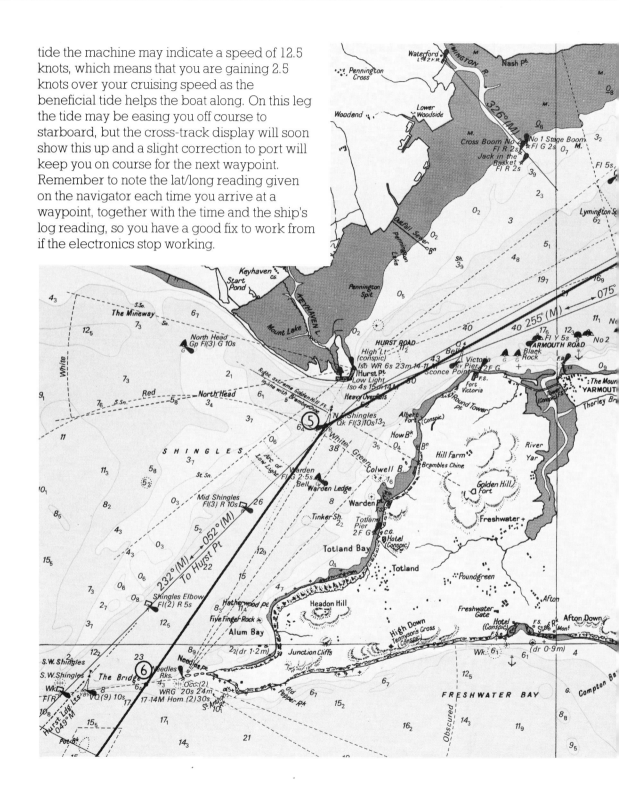

## THE LONG HAUL

Once round the point off the Needles light you will be heading out into the English Channel on course for Alderney some 63 miles away. The tide will be flowing down-Channel, and as in the Solent a cross-track error will start to show on the display. As before, the simple solution is to note the bearing shown to the waypoint off Alderney (waypoint seven) and check it against your COG (course-over-ground). The bearing should be 206 degrees and your COG could be 211 degrees, so the difference is five degrees. This is subtracted from the bearing of the waypoint because the tide is flowing from port to starboard. The waypoint bearing is 206 degrees so when the five-degree difference between it and the COG is subtracted we are left with a course to steer of 201 degrees. The tide flowing in the English Channel is never constant in velocity or direction so further slight course adjustments will have to be made. This usually amounts to a slight course change every half-hour or so to maintain steady progress with full compensation for tide, leeway and differing boatspeeds.

It is imperative that a regular fix of position is plotted on the chart together with the time and log reading. Look at the waypoint display and note the bearing and distance from the next waypoint. This is easy to remember and far easier to plot on a heaving chart table than a lat/long position. It is absolutely identical to the lat/long reading, since both are derived from the same calculation in the internal computer.

If you are using a very popular route (such as Needles to Cherbourg) it would be prudent to move your track at least 100 metres to one side of the direct line to reduce the risk of collision with other navigator-equipped vessels following the same track. A modern electronic navigator linked to an autopilot is capable of holding a course with an error of less than 20 metres on each side – so beware.

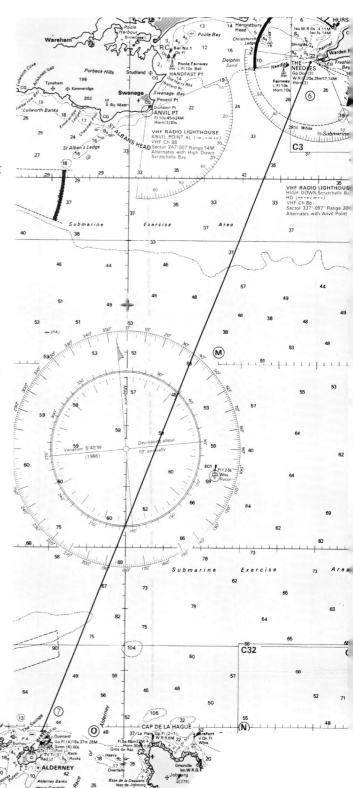

If you are sailing and the wind is uncooperative, forcing you to tack across the Channel, then select a suitable distance either side of the downwind line (see page 36) and tack to it. For example, if you decide to tack five miles either side of the downwind line, sail close-hauled until the cross-track display shows a five-mile error. Then go about and tack back the other way; the error will reduce down to zero then start to increase in the other direction until you reach five miles again. You can then go about once more and repeat the exercise. This method can be used very effectively until you are within eight miles or so of waypoint seven, when you have to decide how to arrive slightly uptide of the waypoint.

Here you can use a slight variation of electronic waypoint sailing. Draw two bearing lines on the chart from a point just uptide of waypoint seven: one line at 251 degrees and the other at 193 degrees. Call up the waypoint display on the navigator and look at the BRG (bearing to waypoint) figure. Continue sailing until the bearing shows 193 degrees, then go about. Keep on the new tack until the bearing shows 251 degrees and go about again; sail back until you get to bearing 193 again and so on. In effect you have created a 'funnel' from waypoint seven which you are tacking into on shorter and shorter legs until you reach the waypoint. Remember that this information from the set takes into account all tidal, leeway and boatspeed differences on any heading.

⇨ **Confidence in your electronic navigation systems allows you to concentrate on the sailing.**

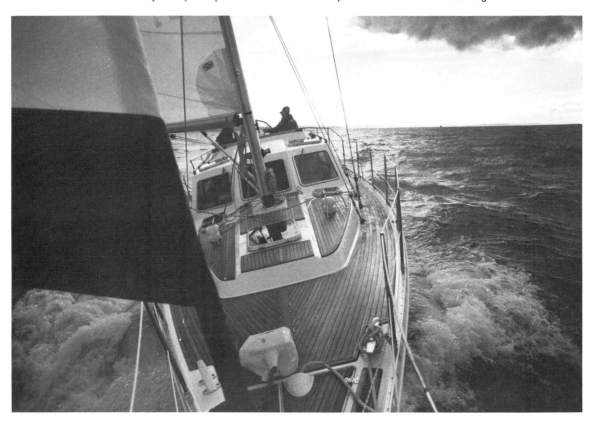

## ARRIVAL AT ALDERNEY

At waypoint seven you turn to port to head for waypoint eight, which is the entrance to Braye Harbour. Be sure to note on the waypoint sheet the position reading your set is showing when you enter the harbour. The next time you are here the harbour may be in thick fog; in such conditions you will want to be able to return to this spot with confidence.

From waypoint eight you enter the harbour and pick up a visitor's mooring for the night. The navigator can now be turned off. The internal battery will remember the position, and all the waypoint information, ready for switch-on the next day. If you own a limited waypoint machine such as the Navstar 300D, Decca/AP MK 2 or the Decca/AP MK 4 its memory capacity will be limited to nine way-

points. So while you are tied up to the mooring, waypoints 10, 11 and 12 can be entered into positions one, two and three (you have passed these points and they are now unwanted). This means that the next waypoint after number nine will be waypoint one and so on. With other machines with large memories the sequence is not a problem and will run through from point one to point 12 without any alterations.

## ALDERNEY TO GUERNSEY

Next day, turn the navigator on just prior to departure to allow the set to lock on to the appropriate chain and settle down. Check the position on the display to ensure that it knows it is in Braye Harbour, then cast off. Motor along the line of mooring buoys and then turn out of

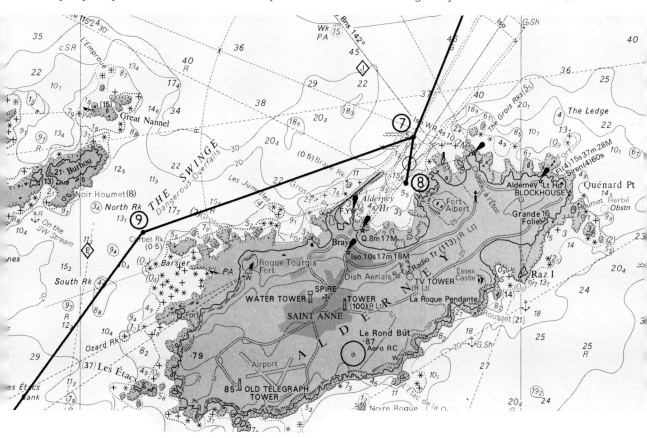

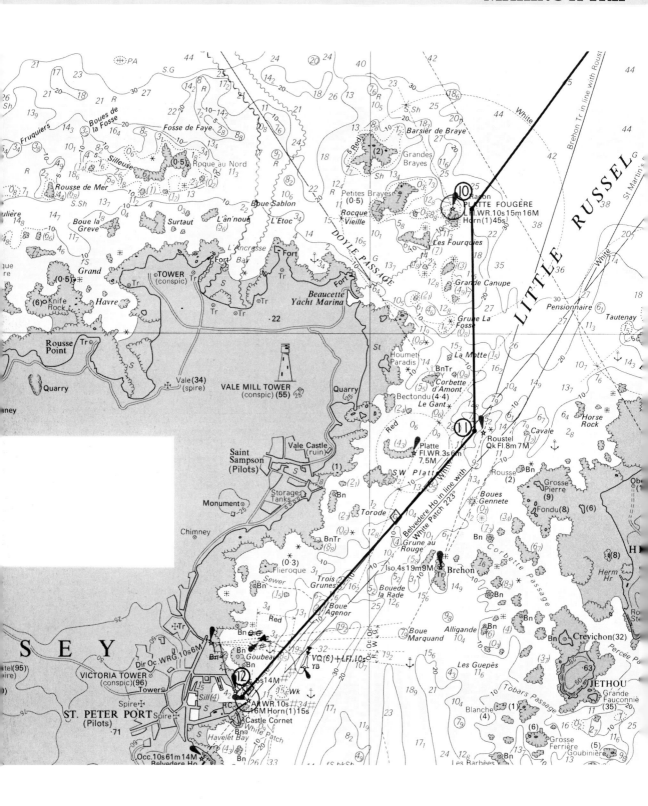

the harbour entrance heading for waypoint seven, the point off Braye Harbour. If you look at the navigator at this stage it will be showing a large cross-track error, indicating that you should turn to port – but if you follow its advice you will hit the harbour wall! The error is showing because the navigator is working on a line directly from your overnight mooring buoy to waypoint seven. So ignore this cross-track error, or reset the machine to zero. On a Navstar 2000D just enter zero followed by ENTER and the error will return to zero. On other machines a simple trick is to turn the navigator off and on. This will force it to re-orientate itself and then it will be working on a direct line from your position to the waypoint.

From waypoint seven set course for waypoint nine. This time you have to keep a strict watch on the cross-track error, because the Swinge channel is not very wide and is flanked by dangerous rocks. When you reach waypoint nine, the point in the Swinge, alter course for waypoint 10 which is off Platte Fougere light on Guernsey. On this leg it is also essential to keep to the track line as the infamous Pierre au Vriac rock lies to starboard of your course and is unmarked. The tides are variable in direction here depending on your start time, so keep a watchful eye on the navigator to allow small course corrections to be made. Use these opportunities to press other buttons on the set such as COG (course-over-ground) and SOG (speed-over-ground), and call up the signal strength display to reassure yourself that the four signals are coming in at acceptable levels.

You can look at the ETA to waypoint to plan your arrival time or prepare for a possible sail change, and of course you must plot your position on the chart at regular intervals.

Waypoint 11 is off the Platte Fougere light, which is left to starboard. The next leg brings you down to Roustel tower, which is left to port, and the final approach to waypoint 12, St Peter Port Harbour entrance. After the relief and thrill of completing the passage do not forget to take a position reading when you are midway between the harbour entrance walls. On a foggy night you will be very grateful that you took this reading, for it will enable you to find your way back in the worst visibility.

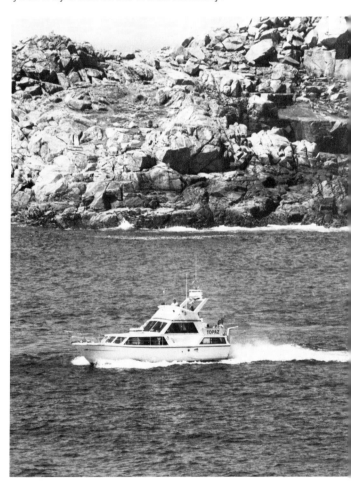

◊ **The rocky shores of the Channel Islands are swept by powerful tides and bristling with off-lying dangers. In such areas the continuous position updates provided by electronic navigation systems are invaluable.**

# 10   Errors: Decca and Loran C

The most common operator error, the east/west longitude mistake, has been mentioned already (see page 21). Normally this is easily spotted if it appears on a waypoint in the middle of a route because it gives bearing and distance figures that are miles out. One advantage of using the waypoint sheet is that you can check each time you turn onto a new waypoint heading to see if the bearing and distance you noted on the sheet correspond to the figures on the navigator. Remember the ancient computer saying 'Garbage in means garbage out'.

## BAD RECEPTION AREAS

On Decca or Loran C systems the sets work out positions using received transmissions, which they calculate as crossed bearings to give a fix. The angle of these bearings to each other is significant. If you were taking bearings with a hand bearing compass you would not take sights on two objects that were very close to each other because the angle of cut would be too acute for accuracy. A similar situation can be found with Decca and Loran C navigation systems, which suffer from bad fix areas called baseline extension areas. In simple terms, if you draw a line on a chart from the master station through each of the slave stations and beyond, there is a bad reception area on the far side of each slave transmitter. In practice this is rarely a problem because the station sites have been carefully chosen so that most of the bad areas are on land. Nevertheless there are one or two that can cause concern. For example, one of the slaves for the SW British Decca chain is on the island of Jersey, and about 20 miles south of the island you can sail into a bad area which is roughly 20 miles across. After you have sailed through it things return to normal and accurate landfalls can be made. This particular area is around the rocky region known as the Minquiers, and it is a fact that not many Decca-type navigators can find the North-east Minquiers Buoy.

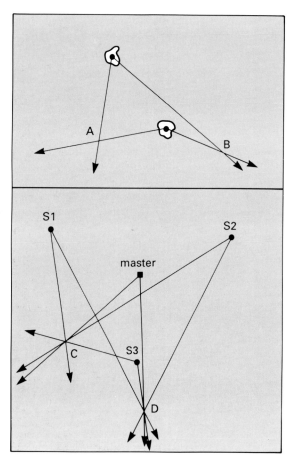

◊  **A sailor using a hand-bearing compass at point A will get a more precise fix than he would at point B, because the position lines have a better angle of cut. In much the same way, an electronic navigator at point C gets a good fix off the nearby master and slave stations. At point D (a baseline extension area) the nearest stations give poor information while the other slaves in the chain (S1 and S2) could well be out of range.**

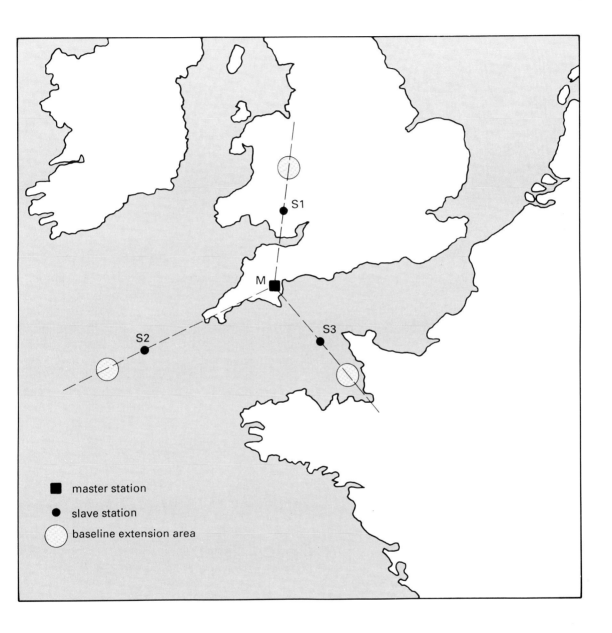

master station

slave station

baseline extension area

◁ Each Decca chain has three baseline extension areas of
poor reception. In the case of the SW British chain, the
northern slave (S1) gives a bad reception area in the Welsh
hills (hardly a problem for the seafarer!) while the western
slave (S2) gives a bad reception area in the open Atlantic
beyond the Scilly Isles, where there is plenty of searoom. But
the southern slave (S3) gives a bad reception area right over
the Minquiers reef south of Jersey. . . .

By studying the Decca and Loran C propagation diagrams in the owners' handbooks you can work out for yourself where these bad areas are and be prepared for problems when you sail into them.

Other areas of bad signals are the points at which the set automatically changes chains (groups of stations) as the boat moves around the coast. When you sail into one of these areas the set will sometimes hunt backwards and forwards trying to determine the best chain or group to operate on. This effect can sometimes be suffered over an area between five and eight miles across. Satellite navigators do not have these problems and will work effectively in all areas, both on land and sea.

## SPOTTING THE PROBLEM

It is possible to spot when a Decca or Loran set is having a struggle to receive good information. The position and cross-track displays on the navigator are updated every few seconds while the other functions such as course-made-good, waypoint bearing and speed are averaged over several minutes. Consequently the cross-track display will start to jump up and down very quickly if there are any signal problems. At the same time a suspect position alarm may activate and the third slave alarm could also join in. As the bearing and course displays are working on a slower average they do not jump around, so it pays to watch them rather than the jittery cross-track information.

Baseline extension areas are here to stay but provided you follow the advice given they will not present a problem. Chain change areas will sometimes give strange results, with jumping cross-track displays and activating alarms. There are a few places where you get both: a baseline extension area coupled with a chain change. One example of the two problems coming together is the area around the Royal Sovereign Light Tower off the south coast of England. Here you have a chain change from 1B to 5B, plus a baseline extension from 5B to contend with.

All low-frequency radio waves are subject to sunrise/sunset effects, and radio transmissions can be unpredictable at these times. So treat Loran and Decca sets with some suspicion when they are operating at dawn and dusk. One way of checking is to call up the display called the 'diamond of error'. This shows two figures for winter and summer. The two figures

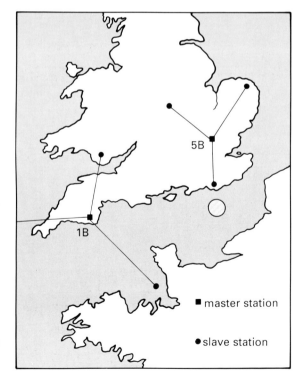

◊ **Just south of the Royal Sovereign light off southern England, a boat travelling east enters a chain change area as the Decca navigator switches from chain 1B to chain 5B. This can cause signal problems that are aggravated by the fact that this is also a baseline extension area from 5B.**

5B

1B

■ master station

● slave station

refer to the size of the diamond formed by lane signals crossing from the two strongest slave stations; in other words the minimum accuracy obtainable by the set at that moment. Generally the figures given are very pessimistic, and much better results can usually be obtained without difficulty. Do not forget the possibility of errors being caused by electrical interference (which has been covered in chapter 1 at length).

## AVOIDING PROBLEMS

Decca-type navigators can be divided into three groups: two-channel sets, four-channel sets and five-channel sets. In simple terms, each transmission from the master or slave station has five pieces of information contained within its signal. Five-channel receivers work with all the information, but these sets are very expensive and are generally used only in aircraft where speeds over 200 knots are normal. The four-channel sets are using about 85 per cent of the available information, whereas two-channel sets use only 25 per cent of the total. What this means to you as a boat owner is that in the event of poor reception, because you are in a bad area or operating at extreme range, a two-channel set will give inferior performance or stop working altogether.

Currently the AP/Decca MK3, the Shipmate 4100 and the Navstar Dinghy D are the three most popular two-channel sets; nearly all other models are full four channel units.

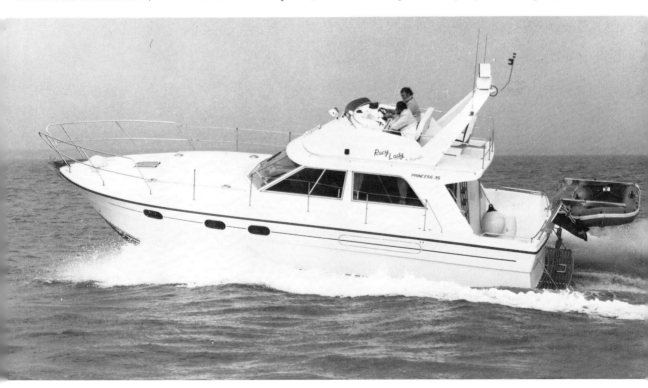

▽ **The author at the helm, watching his cross-track error (or is he reminiscing about that party the other night?)**

# 11   Errors: GPS and Transit

The GPS Navstar satellite system is so new that at the time of writing very few errors have been experienced. At present the GPS coverage is giving around 22 hours per day and during this period the errors experienced by the author have been remarkably small.

Working at speeds of up to 40 knots, the position information has been accurate to less than three metres and remains unaffected by sunrise/sunset, weather conditions, electrical storms and shipborne interference. Small amounts of electrical noise can be introduced via the power supply, but so far this has not affected the operation of the GPS set.

For security reasons the GPS system may be deliberately downgraded to provide 'selective availability' in certain critical areas such as busy ports. It is said that this will reduce the accuracy to roughly 100 metres. At the time of writing, however, the fixes are accurate to within a few metres.

## TRANSIT

Satellite navigators working on the Transit system are more prone to errors. The basic set-up information the set needs is GMT or UTC time, an approximate position and the aerial height above sea level. From then on just the ship's course and speed are required. The ship's heading can be entered manually or via a heading sensor, as described in Chapter 2. The boatspeed can also be entered manually or via a log sending unit. Of the three figures the speed is the one that can have the most serious effect on fix accuracy: a difference of one knot can alter the fix elevation by approximately 0.2 miles.

The elevation of each satellite can affect the fix accuracy. Those lower than 10 degrees or

higher than 75 degrees to the horizon are automatically dismissed by the internal computer, but fixes obtained from satellite passes near these elevations can be up to five miles out. All transit sets have some sort of grading system for fix quality and accuracy, and this enables the operator to dismiss the more dubious figures. Shipmate sets have a simple alphabetic grading from A to E: 'A' fixes are accurate to within 100 metres and 'E' fixes are accurate to within a few miles. Other sets use a star grading – the more stars a fix has, the better – and some use elevation figures.

The author has a Transit Satnav running 24 hours a day connected to a printer. The average number of fixes in 24 hours is 31, and the accuracy of these can be summarised as follows:

- 12 fixes accurate to within 100 metres
- 9 fixes accurate to within 500 metres
- 4 fixes accurate to within 1000 metres
- 2 fixes accurate to within 5000 metres
- 4 fixes accurate to within 10,000 metres

These are average figures for winter in the south of England. Remember that you will experience gaps of up to three hours without any fixes at all. Conversely there are times when you can obtain three top-grade fixes in one hour. The DR system will fill in the gaps as you travel along, but the quality of a dead reckoning position is limited by the accuracy of the last fix.

◊   **The limited accuracy of the Transit Satnav system is no problem offshore, but owing to the extended intervals between fixes, and the poor quality of some of them, it is not recommended for inshore navigation.**

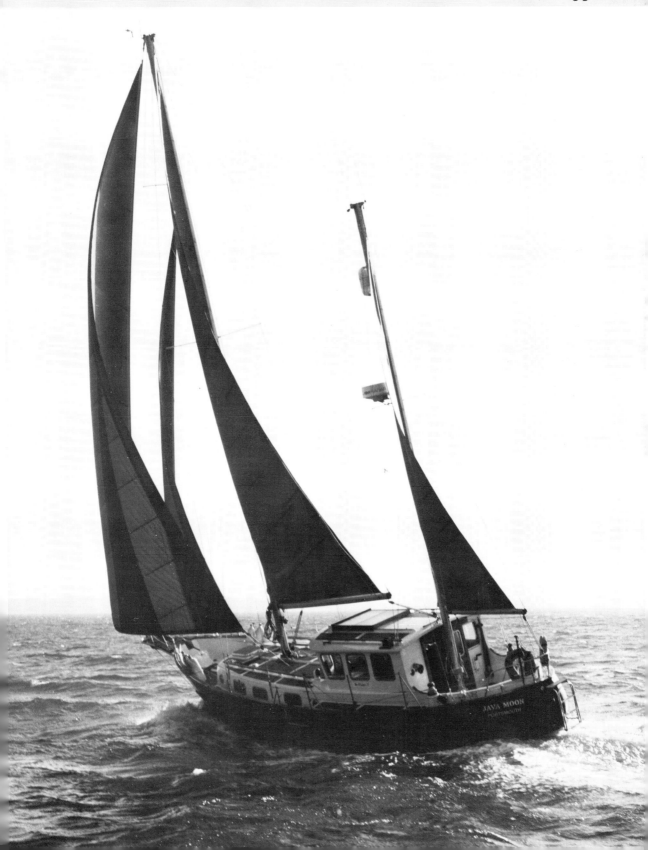

# 12  Advanced Functions

This chapter really concerns the owners of Decca and Loran systems who, once they are familiar with the operation of their sets, may wish to make better use of some of the more advanced functions available. In normal circumstances these functions work automatically, but if necessary they can be overridden to achieve better results in bad reception conditions such as in baseline extension areas, chain change areas and places where the signals are weak such as the Bay of Biscay.

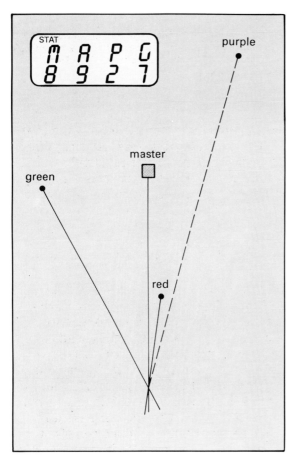

## MANUAL CHAIN SELECTION

Normally the set automatically selects the best chain or group of stations to work with, but there are some circumstances that justify the operator overriding this auto function. For example, if you are half-way across the Bay of Biscay the Decca reception can be very intermittent as the set jumps between the English, French and Spanish chains. One solution is to switch to manual chain selection, and choose the chain that you are going towards. Initially the accuracy obtained may be poor as you are working at the maximum range of the chain, but as the land draws nearer (and good navigation becomes more critical) the signals improve and accurate landfalls can be made. A similar situation can occur along the English south coast around the Royal Sovereign Light Tower. Here there is a chain change area plus a baseline extension area to deal with. The same rule applies: just enter the chain number you are going towards and the set will lock onto that chain; within a few miles it will start giving good information.

If you are in a baseline extension area and your navigator is giving intermittent results you can mask out the third slave station on some sets. To do this you first call up the signal strength display; if one slave is showing a very poor figure then it is probably worthwhile eliminating it from the computer calculation.

◊  Here the 'status' display is indicating a poor signal from the purple slave, which may be confusing the issue. Sometimes masking out the slave station concerned will eliminate errors and result in a better fix.

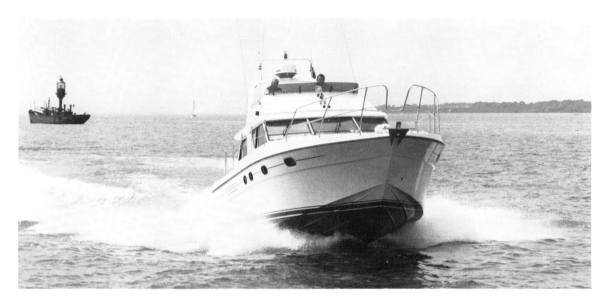

The danger of these override functions is that they stay active in the set long after the fault has disappeared. If you change *any* of the automatic functions to manual then place a large sticker near the set to remind you to reset it to normal after you have passed through the problem area. The author found one yachtsman who sailed for years off the east coast of England with his Decca navigator working reliably and accurately at all times – except during his annual cruise down to the Channel Islands. Here his Decca never worked at all, but when he sailed back up to his home waters the machine worked perfectly again. His problem was simple: the set was switched to manual chain selection for the eastern chain. When he came south he simply ran out of transmitter range.

## CORRECTED POSITION

All Decca and Loran C sets have a corrected position input facility. This is used only if you know *exactly* what your position is: you enter this into the set and from then on the lat/long position has this correction applied to it. This

⌖ **If you know exactly where you are you can correct the navigator by entering a corrected position. This correction is then automatically applied thereafter, but it is of limited value in practice.**

function is of use only over a very limited area because by moving just a couple of miles the correction factor could change. The best method is to note the position the *set* is giving and always use that reading when you want to return to the same spot.

## LINES OF POSITION

Some units on the market can give positions in LOP (lines of position) format. To use this type of output you will need a Decca or Loran C lattice chart. This was the original method employed by the system before yacht-type navigators were introduced with computers that convert LOP readings to lat/long notation. Some fishermen still use LOP information, but very few yachtsmen bother with the extra charts necessary and the added complication of dealing with two sets of position coordinates.

# 13   The theory

The Second World War provided the impetus for many technological developments that are now in daily use all over the world, and among these were two systems designed to ensure pinpoint navigation at night or in poor visibility. In the USA a system of radio navigation called Loran A was developed for use by the armed forces. Meanwhile the British Decca company was developing its own system of night-time radio navigation.

Loran A was succeeded by an upgraded version some years ago called Loran C. The system operates with master and secondary (slave) stations transmitting radio pulses at precise time intervals relative to each other. The further away your receiver is from a station,

the longer it takes for the pulse to be 'heard'. By carefully measuring the time difference between the signals from each of the stations in the group, the receiver can determine its position relative to that group.

The Decca system also uses groups of radio stations, each known as a 'chain'. These transmit continuous wave signals which, at the outset, are accurately kept in phase between the master and slave stations. The receiver listens to the master station and one slave, and can calculate a position line by measuring the degree to which the received signals are in or out of phase. By automatically cross-checking with another pair of stations the machine can produce an accurate fix.

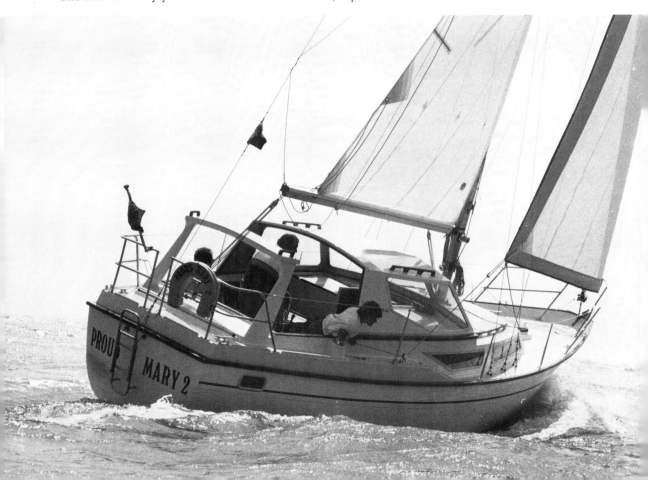

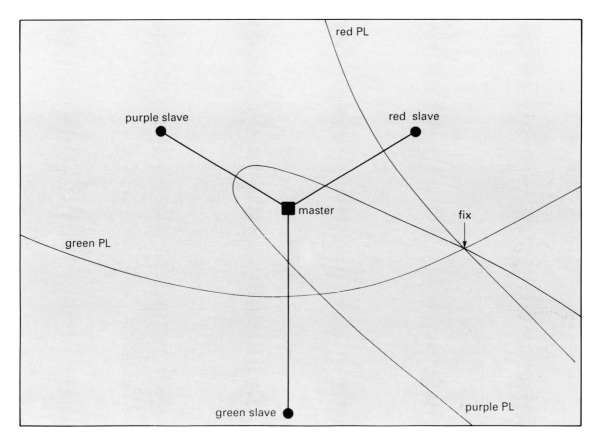

red PL

purple slave

red slave

green PL

master

fix

purple PL

green slave

⌐ Before the appearance of machines with lat/long output, Decca positions were plotted using hyperbolic position lines which correspond to the signals generated by the transmitting stations. The lattice charts used for such plotting are covered with a network of these curved lines, and for most people the problems of working with them negate any theoretical advantages.

## SATNAV

The Transit satellite system was first switched on by the US Coastguard during 1964 for military purposes only. It was opened up for civilian use during 1967 when the first 'yacht' navigators appeared on the market. It consists of six satellites, each orbiting the Earth every 107 minutes.

Since the original units were sent into space

some 'Nova' models have been added to the system and these are capable of being steered with the aid of little thruster rockets. This has allowed the orbits to be adjusted to give more even coverage, with less time between fixes.

The system makes use of the Doppler Effect, in which the frequency of a radio transmission alters depending on whether the transmitter (the satellite) is approaching or leaving the receiver. The set has a very accurate internal clock; by using this, and knowing the exact speed of the satellite, it can work out the rate of approach. In very simple terms it takes a running fix on a passing satellite as it goes by, then records the information for the operator to recall later.

The GPS (Global Positioning System) is similar but makes use of more satellites. The complete system will consist of 21 satellites each rotating in a fixed orbit. Full three-dimensional coverage giving latitude, longitude and height will require at least 18 satellites, but we seafarers need only two-dimensional coverage giving latitude and longitude – for which 12 satellites will be sufficient. They will orbit the Earth in just under 12 hours, and are arranged so that at least four satellites are above the horizon at any one time, wherever you are in the world.

The principle of operation is similar to that of the Transit system, but with more satellites in view the position updates are virtually instantaneous and remarkably accurate. The American space shuttle disaster put back the completion of the system by several years, but the latest information suggests that the 24-hour two-dimensional service will be operating early in the year 1991.

At the moment GPS sets are expensive (at least five times the price of Transit sets) and because of the more complex hardware they may never be available at the low prices of Decca or Loran C equipment, but as more manufacturers swing into action prices will fall and should be affordable by the time the system is fully operational.

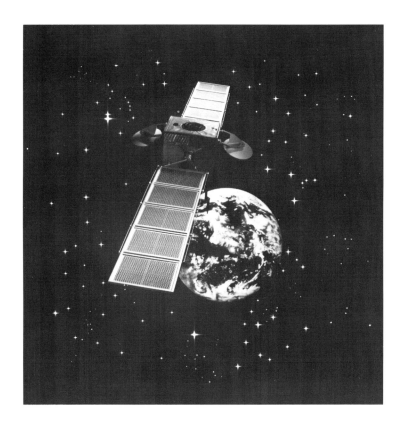

# Glossary

**Auto-locate** A facility that enables an electronic navigator to find its starting position automatically.

**Baseline extension area** An area roughly 20 miles across, on the extension of the line passing through the master station and a slave station, where position-fixing is suspect owing to poor signals.

**Chain** A group of Decca transmitting stations consisting of a master station and three slaves.

**Chain change area** An area between two Decca chains that may cause problems with some navigators as they switch to and fro between chains.

**Chain selection** A manual over-ride facility, allowing the operator to switch to a different Decca chain and avoid the problems associated with chain change areas.

**Corrected position input** A correction that can be keyed into a Decca or Loran set if the known position differs from the indicated position. Once keyed in, the correction is applied to all subsequent positions irrespective of local anomalies.

**Course-made-good (CMG)** The actual course followed by the boat under the influence of tide and leeway, rather than its compass heading.

**Course-over-ground (COG)** See Course-made-good.

**Cross-track error** Your position relative to the track line between two waypoints, displayed on the machine as the distance you have strayed to one side of the track.

**Dead reckoning (DR)** A system of finding a rough position by calculating forward from the last good fix, using speed and direction information. In Transit satellite navigators, the calculation is done automatically.

**Deviation** The error induced in a compass by ship-borne magnetic influences.

**Great circle (GC)** The shortest route between two points on the globe, which may appear as a curved course on charts with normal projection.

**Ground plate** A metal plate attached to the hull below water level, which when connected to the earth wire of electronic equipment ensures a good connection to 'earth'.

**Heading** The compass course and apparent direction of sailing (see Course-made-good).

**Heading reference unit** In essence, a compass that is electronically connected to a Transit satellite navigator to supply heading information for DR calculations.

**Interface** A signal output that is tailored to suit the requirements of a particular type of ancillary unit such as a printer or autopilot.

**Lattice chart** A special chart showing the lines of position radiated by Decca or Loran stations, now made redundant (for most purposes) by modern sets that electronically convert the information into lat/long co-ordinates.

**Leeway** The amount by which any boat drifts under the influence of the wind.

**Line of position (LOP)** A line used on a lattice chart to determine position.

**Repeat factor** The practice of recording the co-ordinates of a well-defined waypoint (such as a buoy) as displayed by the electronic navigator, rather than as indicated on the chart. This takes account of any local errors in the system, and improves navigation accuracy when returning to the same spot.

**Rhumb line (RL)** A direct line between two points, as marked on a normal chart.

**Speed-made-good (SMG)** The actual speed made by the boat relative to the sea bed, rather than its speed through the water.

**Speed-over-ground (SOG)** See Speed-made-good.

**Speed reference unit** An electronic log that sends information to a Transit satellite navigator for use in DR calculations.

**Status** On some sets, this is the title given to the display that indicates the strength of the signals being received.

**Track** In the context of electronic navigation, the direct route between two waypoints.

**Variation** The difference between true north and magnetic north, which varies from place to place.

**Waypoint** A point selected on the chart which is used as a 'goal' for navigation purposes. The electronic navigator will guide the boat in a straight line until it reaches the waypoint.

| ROUTE: | | | | DATE: | |
|---|---|---|---|---|---|

| NO. | DESCRIPTION | LAT. | LONG. | DIS. | BRG. |
|---|---|---|---|---|---|
| | READING AT WAYPOINT: | | | | |
| | LOG READING AT WAYPOINT: | | TIME AT WAYPOINT: | | |
| | READING AT WAYPOINT: | | | | |
| | LOG READING AT WAYPOINT: | | TIME AT WAYPOINT: | | |
| | READING AT WAYPOINT: | | | | |
| | LOG READING AT WAYPOINT: | | TIME AT WAYPOINT: | | |
| | READING AT WAYPOINT: | | | | |
| | LOG READING AT WAYPOINT: | | TIME AT WAYPOINT: | | |
| | READING AT WAYPOINT: | | | | |
| | LOG READING AT WAYPOINT: | | TIME AT WAYPOINT: | | |
| | READING AT WAYPOINT: | | | | |
| | LOG READING AT WAYPOINT: | | TIME AT WAYPOINT: | | |
| | READING AT WAYPOINT: | | | | |
| | LOG READING AT WAYPOINT: | | TIME AT WAYPOINT: | | |
| | READING AT WAYPOINT: | | | | |
| | LOG READING AT WAYPOINT: | | TIME AT WAYPOINT: | | |
| | READING AT WAYPOINT: | | | | |
| | LOG READING AT WAYPOINT: | | TIME AT WAYPOINT: | | |

# THE WAYPOINT SHEET

This waypoint sheet has been designed as a blank for photocopying. there is space for nine waypoints on each sheet (the maximum capacity of machines with small waypoint memories), but by taking several copies you can record the details of as many waypoints as you like, and file them for future reference.

### Route and date
Fill these in if you are using the sheet to record the waypoints of a particular voyage.

### Waypoint number
For a voyage, the number of each waypoint should correspond to the route or sailplan – that is, the order in which they are entered into the navigator. So waypoint one is the first to be reached on the trip, waypoint two the second, and so on.

If you are using the sheets as a filing system you may prefer to number the waypoints by a different system, and alter the numbers to suit your sailplan when you transfer them to the navigator.

### Description
Enter the name of the waypoint if it has one; for example 'St Peter Port harbour entrance'. Otherwise, identify the position as best you can, and add any distinguishing marks that may help you recognise the waypoint when you get there; for example 'Castle Point Buoy, red can'.

### Lat and long
The top two co-ordinates should represent the position of the waypoint as indicated on the chart.

### Distance
Fill in the distance of each waypoint from the last, as measured on the chart.

### Bearing
Under this heading, fill in the bearing of each waypoint from the last.

### Reading at waypoint
The lower two co-ordinates are filled in as you reach each identifiable waypoint (such as a buoy), using the figures on the navigator display. If the system is not working with complete accuracy you will have to steer 'off-course' to reach the buoy, and as a result this second set of co-ordinates will be different from those entered into the machine. If you want to return to the same spot, enter this second set; the machine will then take you straight to the waypoint, every time.

### Log reading at waypoint
Read the log when you reach the waypoint and enter the figure here. This will help you keep track of your position.

### Time at waypoint
Note the time when you pass the waypoint. If the electronics pack up, the time and log reading will enable you to work out a current dead-reckoning position.

# Also published by Fernhurst Books

Sailing: A Beginner's Manual    *John Driscoll*
Racing: A Beginner's Manual    *John Caig & Tim Davison*
Sailing the Mirror    *Roy Partridge*
Mirror Racing    *Guy Wilkins*
Topper Sailing    *John Caig*
The Laser Book    *Tim Davison*
Laser Racing    *Ed Baird*
The Catamaran Book    *Brian Phipps*
Boardsailing: A Beginner's Manual    *John Heath*


**Sail to Win**

Tactics    *Rodney Pattisson*
Dinghy Helming    *Lawrie Smith*
Dinghy Crewing    *Julian Brooke-Houghton*
Wind Strategy    *David Houghton*
Tuning Your Dinghy    *Lawrie Smith*
The Rules in Practice    *Bryan Willis*
Tides and Currents    *David Arnold*
Boatspeed – Supercharging your hull, foils and gear    *Rodney Pattison*
Sails    *John Heyes*
The Winning Mind – Strategies for successful sailing    *John Whitmore*


**Yachting**

Weather at Sea    *David Houghton*
Inshore Navigation    *Tom Cunliffe*
Coastal and Offshore Navigation    *Tom Cunliffe*
Celestial Navigation    *Tom Cunliffe*
Marine VHF Operation    *Michael Gale*
Heavy Weather Cruising    *Tom Cunliffe*
A Small Boat Guide to the Rules of the Road    *John Mellor*
Yacht Skipper    *Robin Aisher*
Yacht Crewing    *Malcolm McKeag*
Tuning Yachts and Small Keelboats    *Lawrie Smith*
Motor Boating    *Alex McMullen*
Boat Engines    *Dick Hewitt*
Children Afloat    *Pippa Driscoll*
The Beaufort Scale Cookbook    *June Raper*
Knots and Splices    *Jeff Toghill*
A Small Boat Guide to Radar    *Tim Bartlett*